CREATING A CULTURE OF Wellness

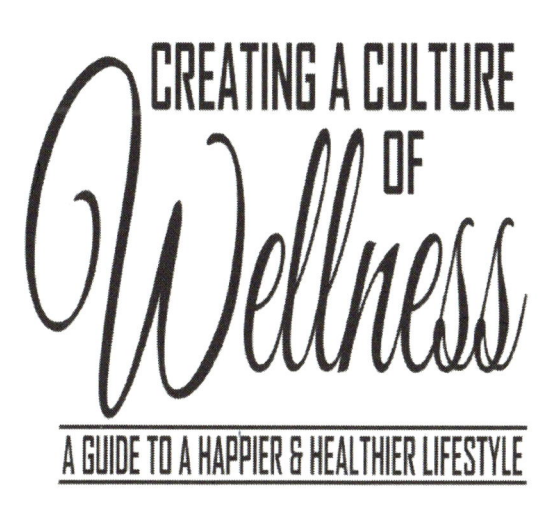

A GUIDE TO A HAPPIER & HEALTHIER LIFESTYLE

Victor Romano, EdD

Contributing Author:
Jennifer Lee

Copyright © 2013
All rights reserved

ISBN: 1492839442
ISBN-13: 978-1492839446

About the Authors

Dr. Victor Romano has more than ten years of experience managing and developing wellness programs for private businesses and nonprofit organizations. He currently is the Director of Wellness, Coordinator of Applied Health Research, and Adjunct Professor at Johnson C. Smith University. His most recent work in partnership with his local health department won the national 'Faith and Community Health Excellence Award' from the US Department of Health and Human Services.

Dr. Romano holds a doctorate in education with a concentration in wellness. He also holds a master's degree in exercise science and health promotion, and a bachelor's degree in exercise and sports studies. In addition, Dr. Romano has multiple certifications in the health and fitness.

Jennifer Lee has spent her career educating children in health and physical education. With particular interests in nutrition and physical education and activity, she taught about healthy food alternatives and the importance of exercise. She is currently working with youth on a Seed-to-Feed program that teaches children about healthy eating, growing food, and sustainability.

She received her Bachelor's Degree in Physical Education from Johnson C. Smith University and her Master's degree in Sport Studies from High Point University.

Introduction

Traditional medicine relies on a reactive approach to healthcare. Disease and medical issues are dealt with after they develop into problems. An increasing number of health professionals and individuals argue this line of thinking is outdated, expensive, and ineffective. Instead of simply treating disease as it emerges, we should instead focus on preventing health problems from developing at all. This paradigm shift forms the basis of the wellness movement.

Wellness takes a holistic approach to health, a fact many "wellness" books forget. Books promoting wellness often have very specific topics: diet, exercise, specific health conditions, or spirituality issues. These are all important aspects of wellbeing, but only parts of the greater holistic whole.

In *Creating a Culture of Wellness*, Dr. Victor Romano helps readers develop a multidimensional approach to wellness, encouraging positive physical, mental, and emotional lifestyle changes. The authors describes seven dimensions of wellness, each equally important to living a happy and healthy lifestyle. They discusses the importance of wellness as it applies to emotional, environmental, intellectual, occupational, physical, social, and spiritual issues. No one of these core areas is more or less important than the others, but when one is out of balance, it affects the other six.

Creating a Culture of Wellness introduces and explains core concepts of wellness in accessible, easily understood language. The final chapters of the book provide helpful data, designed to enhance well-being and improve health.

How important is wellness? The US Centers for Disease Control and Prevention estimates half of all deaths among people sixty-five years of age or younger result from unhealthy lifestyle choices. Embracing holistic wellness helps ensure you live a long, happy, and healthy life.

Table of Contents

CHAPTER 1 Pg. 1
Introducing You to Wellness

CHAPTER 2 Pg. 7
Emotional Wellness

CHAPTER 3 Pg. 27
Environmental Wellness

CHAPTER 4 Pg. 40
Intellectual Wellness

CHAPTER 5 Pg. 54
Occupational Wellness

CHAPTER 6 Pg. 69
Physical Wellness

CHAPTER 7 Pg. 87
Social Wellness

CHAPTER 8 Pg. 102
Spiritual Wellness

HELPFUL INFORMATION Pg. 117

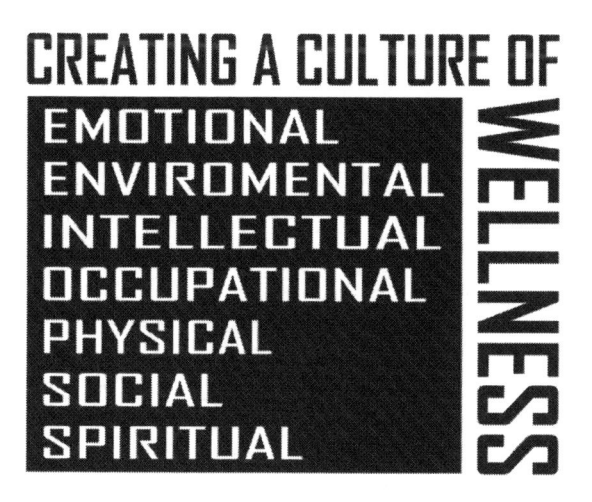

CREATING A CULTURE OF WELLNESS

EMOTIONAL
ENVIROMENTAL
INTELLECTUAL
OCCUPATIONAL
PHYSICAL
SOCIAL
SPIRITUAL

Chapter 1

Wellness represents the positive aspects of all the different dimensions that can help expand your potential to live and work effectively. Wellness is possible for everyone, regardless of whether or not you have a diagnosed disease. In fact, the term "Quality of Life" is used often when referring to a person's state of wellness.

What does wellness mean to you? Wellness is more than being free from illness. Wellness is a dynamic process of change and growth. There are many interrelated dimensions of wellness: physical, emotional, intellectual, spiritual, social, environmental, and occupational. Each dimension is equally vital in the pursuit of optimum health.

The seven dimension model used in this book explains the importance and the interrelation of a healthy lifestyle within the multidimensional domain within your life. Creating a Culture of Wellness is using all of the multi-dimensional aspects of wellness to live a happier and healthier lifestyle. Imagine the seven dimensions of Health mentioned above are parts of a wheel. Just like a car, when one wheel is worn or deflated, the whole car will not work properly and wouldn't drive efficiently anywhere, at least not very quickly. You will be constantly adjusting your steering wheel to the left or right. But, if all the parts of the wheel were equally "inflated", you would find that "driving through life" would become much smoother and more enjoyable.

Generations of people have viewed health simply as the absence of disease. That view largely prevails today; the word health typically refers to the overall condition of a person's body or mind and to the presence or absence of illness or injury. Wellness is a relatively new concept that expands our idea of health. Beyond the simple presence or absence of disease, wellness refers to optimal health and vitality—to living life to its fullest. Although we use the words health and wellness interchangeably, there are two important differences between them:

Health
Health can be determined or influenced by factors beyond your control, such as your genes, age, and family history. For example, consider a 60 year old man with a strong family history of prostate cancer. These factors place this man at a higher than average risk for developing prostate cancer himself.

Wellness
Wellness is largely determined by the decisions you make about how you live. That same 60 year old man can reduce his risk of cancer by eating sensibly, exercising, and having regular screening tests. Even if he develops the disease, he may still rise above its effects to live a rich, meaningful life.

This means choosing not only to care for himself physically but to maintain a positive outlook, keep up his relationships with others, challenge himself intellectually, and nurture other aspects of his life.

Health was originally defined by the World Health Organization in 1946 as "a state of complete physical, mental and social well-being and not merely the absence of disease or infirmity." In 1979, Wellness was created from this idea and has been known to have five main domains: social, emotional, physical, intellectual, and spiritual. Even today, these five domains are still recognized. More recently, researchers have started to add domains to the five core domains, such as occupational and environmental. Over the past 20 years, researchers, foundations, community-based organizations (such as YMCAs), private fitness facilities, and government agencies have designed and implemented a broad range of innovative health promotion and disease prevention programs using multiple domains of wellness. Many of these programs have shown to be effective, resulting in a positive impact on a participant's and a community's overall wellness.

When it comes to striving for wellness, most differences among people are insignificant. We all need to exercise, eat well, and manage stress. We all need to know how to protect ourselves from heart disease, cancer, sexually transmitted diseases, and injuries.

But some of our differences, both as individuals and as members of groups, do have implications for wellness. Some of us, for example, have grown up with eating habits that increase our risk of obesity or heart disease. Some of us have inherited predispositions for certain health problems, such as osteoporosis or high cholesterol levels. These health-related differences among individuals and groups can be biological, determined genetically, or cultural, acquired as patterns of behavior through daily interactions with family, community, and society. Many health conditions are a function of biology and culture combined.

Every person is an individual with her or his own unique genetic endowment as well as unique experiences in life. However, many of these influences are shared with others of similar genetic and cultural backgrounds. Information about group similarities relating to wellness issues can be useful; for example, it can alert people to areas that may be of special concern for them and their families. Wellness-related differences among groups can be described along several dimensions, including:

Gender
Men and women have different life expectancies and different incidences of many diseases, including heart disease, cancer, and osteoporosis. Men have higher rates of death from injuries, suicide, and homicide; women are at greater risk for Alzheimer's disease and depression. Men and women also differ in body composition and certain aspects of physical performance.

Race and Ethnicity
A genetic predisposition for a particular health problem can be linked to race or ethnicity as a result of each group's relatively distinct history. Diabetes is more prevalent among individuals of Native American or Latino heritage, for example, and African Americans have higher rates of hypertension. Racial or ethnic groups may also vary in other ways that relate to wellness: traditional diets; patterns of family and interpersonal relationships; and attitudes toward using tobacco, alcohol, and other drugs, to name just a few.

Income and Education

Inequalities in income and education are an underlying reason for many of the health disparities among Americans. People with low incomes (low socioeconomic status, or SES) and less education have higher rates of injury and many diseases, are more likely to smoke, and have less access to health care. Poverty and low educational attainment are far more important predictors of poor health than any racial or ethnic factor.

A lifestyle based on good choices and healthy behaviors maximizes quality of life. It helps people avoid disease, remain strong and fit, and maintain their physical and mental health as long as they live. A positive sense of wellness involves making conscious decisions to control risk factors that contribute to disease or injury. Age and family history are risk factors you cannot control. Behaviors such as smoking, exercising, and eating a healthy diet are well within your control.

As you may already know from experience, changing an unhealthy habit can be harder than it looks. When you begin to change your behavior, it may seem like too much work at first. But as you make progress, you will gain confidence. You will also experience the benefits of wellness: more energy, greater vitality, deeper feelings of appreciation and curiosity, and a higher quality of life.

If you begin return to old habits, don't give up. Relapse can be demoralizing, but it is not the same as failure; failure means stopping before you reach your goal and never changing your target behavior. During the early stages of the change process, it's a good idea to plan for relapse so you can avoid guilt and self-blame and get back on track quickly. Follow these steps:

Forgive yourself
A single setback isn't the end of the world, but abandoning your efforts to change could have negative effects on your life.

Give yourself credit for your progress
Use successes as motivation to continue.

Move on
Learn from your relapse and use that knowledge to deal with your potential setbacks in the future.

Once you are committed to making a change, it's time to put together your plan of action. The following chapters will describe each dimension of wellness in-depth. This will assist you in creating your personal Culture of Wellness.

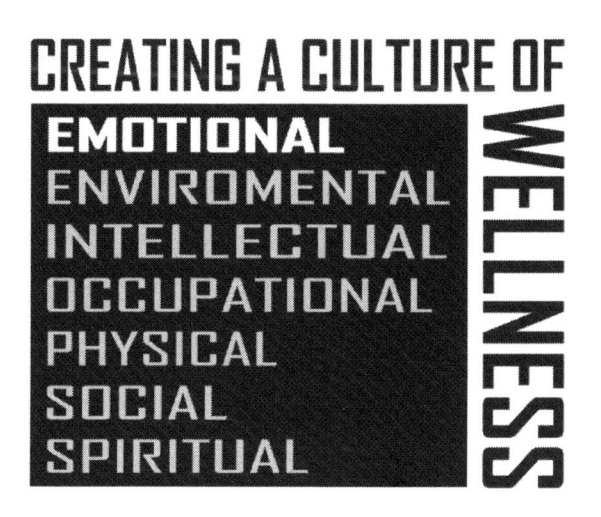

CREATING A CULTURE OF
EMOTIONAL
ENVIROMENTAL
INTELLECTUAL
OCCUPATIONAL
PHYSICAL
SOCIAL
SPIRITUAL
WELLNESS

Chapter 2

| Self-Awareness | Happiness | Anger | Fear |
| Expression of Emotion | Independence | Love |

Emotional wellness is a dynamic state that fluctuates frequently with your other six dimensions of wellness. Being emotionally well is typically defined as possessing the ability to feel and express human emotions such as happiness, sadness, and anger. It means having the ability to love and be loved and achieving a sense of fulfillment in life. Emotional wellness encompasses optimism, self-esteem, self-acceptance, and the ability to share feelings.

Emotional Wellness for adults includes experiencing and expressing a wide range of feelings, developing abilities to cope with life's occurrences through giving and receiving support and learning to trust and rely on one's ability to deal with any situation. Emotional maturity allows us to develop meaningful connections with others and to acknowledge a level of interdependence. Emotional balance allows for diverse reactions to life events while maintaining an ability to function within cultural societies. Emotional wellness enables us to live fully engaged lives that can be shared intimately with others who are important to us.

SELF-AWARENESS

Self-awareness is a way for us to explore our individual personalities, value systems, beliefs, natural inclinations, and tendencies. Because we are all different in the way we react to situations, learn, and process information, it's helpful to spend time in self-reflection to gain a better insight into ourselves. But, why is self-awareness important? Self-awareness is important because when we have a better understanding of who we truly are we are empowered to make changes and to build on our areas of strength as well as identify areas where we would like to make improvements. Self-awareness is the first step towards setting goals for ourselves.

Do you really know yourself? it is good to know your strengths and weaknesses, your most effective learning methods, your preferred communication styles, also to know where you are, where you are going and why. Understanding this will go a long way to self-awareness. Know yourself and you will find it much easier to establish meaningful relationships and develop strong team.

Awareness is a powerful tool. When used the right way it will undo much of the harm we create by lying or creating false beliefs. Much of our behavior stems from unconscious beliefs or patterns. As long as our behaviors

> **"As you become more clear about who you really are, you'll be better able to decide what is best for you - the first time around."**
> *- Oprah Winfrey -*

remain unconscious, we are a slave to them. Without an objective awareness of our unconscious desires or behavior we are powerless to alter them, even when they cause us pain again and again. Self-awareness helps us cut through our own thoughts and actions like a knife. For instance, we say we want to be healthy and live a long life but our behavior might be the total opposite. Awareness is seeing the truth about our behavior, not listening to our excuses or accepting denials. A keener understanding of our behavior is the first step in changing our behavior.

Awareness comes in many forms and levels, and for all we know, each of us has a unique experience of it. For instance, some people experience it through mindfulness, which creates a heightened sense of being. Someone who is mindful may experience sensations inside and outside the body and mind more powerfully than others. Self-awareness can be taught, it can be learned, it can be discovered, but probably can't ever be arrived at. In other words, it's a gradual unpeeling where you never get to the core. There is always something lurking behind current revelations. No one can ever be supremely aware, just more aware than others or more aware than they were yesterday.

Cultivating self-awareness requires the following qualities to be successful:

Be brutally honest with yourself
Without honesty we will be easily fooled by our own self-deceptions.

Be focused on the issue at hand
Without focus we will quickly lose the thread.

Have the determination to see it through
Persistence will win in the end.

Have perspective
Don't let small issues be blown out of proportion.

Be observant and vigilant
I liken it to reserving a part of my mind that looks over my shoulder and watches me.

Be curious
It helps keep us free from judgment. The point isn't to judge ourselves but to just notice and bear witness as objectively as possible.

Trust your feelings
Rather than analyze our actions, which tend to play into the imaginations of our mind, we need to lead with our feelings.

The results of your efforts at becoming more self-aware build authenticity within you. Self-awareness leads to self-confidence by building on knowledge of who you are. You won't experience as many anguished decisions or the feeling of being pulled in two directions quite as often. Self-awareness helps create an inventory of your unconscious behaviors and desires. When all your behaviors are totally integrated into your personality you have achieved a state of being comfortable in your own skin.

🌾 HAPPINESS 🌾

Being happy not only feels good but is good for you. Unfortunately, we don't often know what is going to bring us happiness. Researchers suggest that between 35%-50%

of an individual's general level of happiness could be genetic, but the rest is all you. This depends on other things that you think or don't think and that you do or don't do. Have you ever been dependent on others for your own well-being, or always relied on another for your sanity, calmness, love and happiness? People may never meet your expectations, and all that will result in disappointment, distrust and more miserable moments your own life. Don't worry, this means that you are the key to your own happiness!

Once we meet our basic physical needs of food, shelter, and comfort our life becomes about maximizing happiness. The challenge is that we often get lost or turned around on our path. We end up seeking many things believing they will bring us to that emotional state we desire. We may get the things, but not the feeling we want. When you take time to evaluate the direction and priorities it may be wise to consider how your thoughts and beliefs affect your happiness.

We have been conditioned to focus on external factors and have missed the most important element in determining our happiness. Your mind is filled with assumptions, beliefs, and expectations of what will make you happy. These have been collected over years, both consciously, and unconsciously. They affect and even determine our choices in a way that we may not be aware. Hidden assumptions and false beliefs lead you down the road to disappointment, frustration, and other emotional reactions.

True joy is not for the faint of heart. In order to be happy, individuals must be willing to face adversity, discomfort and tragedy with grace and not be defined by it. Genuinely resilient people who present a strong sense of hope, optimism, and belief in life and themselves tend to be happier. I like to define true happiness as a dynamic state of being that comes from the alignment of our passion, purpose, place, and meaning in the world. If we are without purpose (family, home, service), then we seek purpose in elements outside of our control. Happiness comes from what we can control and how we decide to act.

We have often been told that our actions follow our emotions, but in reality it is the other way around, emotions will follow our actions. So the next time you are not feeling happy then go out in the world and create something happy. Offer a service to another, simplify your schedule for appointments of absolute importance, find a plant to nurture, be actively engaged in a good cause, if not for yourself then for someone else. Happiness is a natural reaction to unselfishness, it is a contagious emotion. And that is a contagion worth contracting.

Positive emotions help us to build the resources that lead to happier lives, such as friends, knowledge, better problem solving, and even better health. Even more, they can act as a buffer against stress and help us cope when we face difficulties. Think of it this way, each of us has the absolute freedom to be happy and at the very same time, the liberty to be miserable. Take responsibility for your own lives, and ultimately the joy that comes from it.

ANGER

We all know what anger is, and we've all felt it: whether as a fleeting annoyance or as full-fledged rage. Anger is a completely normal, usually healthy, human emotion. But when it gets out of control and turns destructive, it can lead to problems: problems at work, in your personal relationships, and in the overall quality of your life. And it can make you feel as though you're at the mercy of an unpredictable and powerful emotion.

The instinctive, natural way to express anger is to respond aggressively. Anger is a natural, adaptive response to threats; it inspires powerful, often aggressive, feelings and behaviors, which allow us to fight and to defend ourselves when we are attacked. A certain amount of anger, therefore, is necessary to our survival. On the other hand, we can't physically lash out at every person or object that irritates or annoys us; laws, social norms, and common sense place limits on how far our anger can take us.

Don't let your anger get the best of you though, as even the smallest amount of stress will set off individuals differently and their responses are typically misplaced and overblown. Disorganized anger will often wreak havoc on people's lives by interfering with their relationships, jobs, and even their health.

People express their anger differently. You must be able to work with people on this. You have those that are often verbally abusive or engage in physically aggressive behavior when upset. Then there are the others who don't explode, they hold it in and experience and keep all the anger in their heads.

However, anger is not always a bad thing. Most people see anger as negative because of the way it was communicated and expressed. However, when anger is expressed appropriately it is healthy, healing and transformative and it is also a way of including intimacy, connection and communication in a relationship. The key is being able to learn how to handle and deal with your anger. Anger management based on emotional intelligence skill enhancement may actually be one of the latest and most effective forms of intervention.

Know the things that cause you to get angry
If you're struggling with out-of-control anger, you may be wondering why your fuse is so short. Anger

problems often stem from what you've learned as a child. If you watched others in your family scream, hit each other, or throw things, you might think this is how anger is supposed to be expressed. Traumatic events and high levels of stress can make you more susceptible to anger as well. Learn these stressors so you can begin to find ways to deal with them.

Own up to your anger
When we suffer, we always blame the other person for having made us suffer. We do not realize that anger is, first of all, our business. We are primarily responsible for our anger, but we believe very naively that if we can say something or do something to punish the other person, we will suffer less.

Identify the source of your anger
Big fights often happen over something small, like a dish left out or being ten minutes late. But there's usually a bigger issue behind it. If you find your irritation and anger rapidly rising, ask yourself "What am I really angry about?" Identifying the real source of frustration will help you communicate your anger better, take constructive action, and work towards a resolution.

Think before you speak
In the heat of the moment, it's easy to say something you'll later regret. Take a few moments to collect your thoughts before saying anything, and also allow others involved in the situation to do the same.

Deal with your anger quickly
As soon as you're thinking clearly, express your frustration in an assertive but non-confrontational way. State your concerns and needs clearly and

directly, without hurting others or trying to control them.

Forgive
Angry people feel that anger entitles them to let loose. It's up to other people not to take seriously hurtful things they say or do. After all, they say, they were just angry. They don't get it that other people are legitimately hurt, embarrassed, humiliated, or afraid. But in no way does this give them a free pass during arguments.

Yes, there are a lot of things that make us angry, but the truth is anger is a choice. There are some things that seem impossible not to get angry about, yes. But the length of time that you are angry is up to you. Honestly, no one likes to be around someone who is always in a bad mood or has a hot temper. So how do you lower your anger? Implement this phrase into your life, "Can't Change it." Most of the time, you can't change it! It's done, it happened, and there's nothing you can do to go back and change it. So, you have a choice. Focus on the bad and stay upset, or accept it and move forward. Put acceptance into your stress life. Eventually you may not have one!

🦋 FEAR 🦋

In our busy and complicated lives, our mind must deal with numerous details as we plan and orchestrate our lives. Our mind can shift effortlessly from present reality to past incidents or future possibilities within seconds. When considering our future, whether that future is one hour or ten years away, the mind can creatively project us into any situation it chooses, and often it does. Fear is the result of our mind becoming fixated on images of an undesirable situation we "fear" will happen to us in the future. The effects of this fear are very real, and they have their consequences. It is not just an unpleasant experience to be ignored or accepted stoically. Fear is a very powerful force. Even those of us who understand what scares us can fall within fear's grasp if we are not diligent.

You cannot get "rid" of a fear, you can only become "okay" with a fear – when you become okay with a fear, you have to overcome that fear. If you seek to get rid of a fear you will be entrapped in that fear in some way or another. Once you accept this simple truth that you can't get rid of a fear, you are already working in alignment with reality and hence have a better chance of finding balance/freedom. To become "okay" with a fear is not a technique, it's not some positive affirmation deal, it's not a pointer to try and convince yourself about the okay-ness of a fear, it's actually about the openness to let the fear be, to allow it fully as a thought and a feeling, until you are okay with its presence knowing that fear is an aspect of life.

There is no escaping it either, as fear and the marketing of paranoia and uncertainty have become daily staples in today's culture. Every day there arise new threats to national security manufactured by politicians and fuelled by the public's demand to be protected. History has shown that living in a culture dominated by fear and ignorance can have catastrophic consequences if it is leveraged by the right people. So, the meaning and experience of fear will continually be shaped by cultural and historical factors.

Fear empowers itself over you which creates important implications on your identity, like how we see and understand ourselves. The idea that we are the subject of constant threats has given rise to the concept of generally being 'at risk'. The emergence of this 'at risk' category ruptures the traditional relationship between individual action and the probability of a hazard. To be 'at risk' is no longer just about the probability of some hazard impacting on you; it is also about who you are as a person.

When we learn to see fear in a different light it begins to lose its power over our lives. Fear is generally related to something that has not yet happened and even if it does it probably will not be as extreme as we have thought about in our imagination. By staying focused on fear we generally bring things more quickly into our life experience to feel fearful of. Fear rules the world now but, if we become less fear-based in our own lives, things can change and a happier and more peaceful world will be the result.

Expression of Emotion

You probably know someone who is a master at managing their emotions. They don't get angry in stressful situations. Instead, they have the ability to look at a problem and calmly find a solution. They're excellent decision makers, and they know when to trust their intuition. Regardless of their strengths, however, they're usually willing to look at themselves honestly. They take criticism well, and they know when to use it to improve their performance. People like this have a high degree of emotional maturity. They know themselves very well, and they're also able to sense the emotional needs of others.

We all have different personalities, different wants and needs, and different ways of showing our emotions. Navigating through this all takes tact and cleverness, especially if we hope to succeed in life. This is where managing your emotions becomes important.
Feelings form a basic element of human interaction. Even brief day-to-day encounters involve an exchange of emotion, whether it's a kiss goodbye as your kids catch the school bus, a quick catch-up with a client over lunch, or a friendly nod to a passerby on the street.

How you express feelings is determined by a complex matrix of innate personality traits and tendencies, cultural and familial influences, as well as the context or social setting. The core fundamentals of emotional development are having the ability to identify and understand your own feelings and manage your strong emotions and how you express them.

Just as you have choices about how to interpret an event, you also have options about how to express those feelings you experience. Often we limit the range of our expressive options by erroneously believing that there are only two options: either directly expressing them to someone else (e.g., in a personal confrontation), or "swallowing" the feelings and keeping them to ourselves.

When you "swallow" your feelings, it means that you just are not willing to express them but it also means that you are choosing to deny and deal with your feelings. Emotions process fast. It takes about 100 milliseconds for our brain to react emotionally and about 600 milliseconds for thinking brain to register this reaction. By the time you have already decided that it's better not to get mad or to be sad, your face has already shown your true feelings. The people close to you know the second that there is something going on, then when you say "Oh, nothing is wrong. I am fine." The people close to you know also know that you are shutting them out.

You do it because you don't know what else to do. In actuality, there are many ways to respond to your feelings and express yourself. To some extent, you express a feeling any time your behavior is influenced by that feeling, but the way you express that feeling, and the intensity of that expression can vary widely. It is hard work, but learning to better communicate your emotions could impact your physical and psychological health and improve the quality of relationships in your home and work life.

Now let's discuss the assumption men do not express their emotions... People have the preconceived notion that men simply do not have feelings. This is far from the case. The problem is in the fact that women believe men should feel things the way they do, which they do. The truth is that men just have a harder time processing their feelings. Why? Because men are taught from an early age that they need to be strong and confident, equating emotions at an early age with weakness. Societal expectations have taught men not to display any emotions. This has been a widely spoken about problem in relationships as men tend not to have socially acceptable emotional outlets. They do not want to feel emasculated in front of their peers for caring about someone or something on a deep level.

> *"Emotions live in the background of a man's life and the foreground of a woman's."*
> *- Josh Coleman -*

In general, it is important to become a good observer of your feelings, to accept and value them, and to attend to what they signal to you. Pay attention to how your interpretations and thoughts affect how you feel and also how the lessons learned in your family about emotional expression continue to influence your behavior. When deciding how to express how you feel, give some thought to all of your options. Maybe, give those closest to you a chance to show you that they care, and that they can be there for you by opening up to them.

INDEPENDENCE

The American Revolution is an amazing story for many reasons. During times of great hardship and injustice, great ideas, great principles and great courage brought 13 colonies to break free and form the United States of America. The independence was needed to create a society of the people based on principles of liberty. This was vital for an individual or group to be free.

But how does one become independent? It often begins as a child. From day one, parents take on the role of nurturer for their children while teaching the importance of independence. For those who just became an adult, showing your parents how well they've raised you is a necessary start to establishing independence on your own.

But this generation of young adults has reported feeling like adults later and later in life, usually relating back to overbearing. Parents are becoming less trustworthy of their children saying they have not learned to trust themselves and make their own adult decisions. In other words, if you don't have to grow up, you are not always going to seek that independence. It's much easier to depend on your parents if they will provide your every need, both financially and psychologically.

While it's extremely important to have connections like family, friends, and significant others in your life, it's also good to feel confident doing things on your own! Independence is something everyone should strive for: the ability to be self-sufficient and in charge of their own life.

Making a conscious decision to gain your own independence, make your own decisions and support yourself financially is the first step toward personal independence. When you find yourself contemplating a decision and wondering what mom and dad would do, stop and explore how you feel about the situation. If you lack the skills to exhibit complete independence, now is the time to gain those skills no matter your age.

Here is how:
- ❖ Accept yourself
- ❖ Take control of your own destiny
- ❖ Be confident on your two feet
- ❖ Become emotionally independent
- ❖ Realize and accept that life sometimes is not fair
- ❖ Try not to care what others think
- ❖ Begin on a career path

> *"Children learn more from what you are than what you teach."*
> *- W.E.B. Du Bois -*

Obviously for those who do not desire independence it is not important but for those who value their independence it is important because it means that others have little if any ability to make choices that oppose your goals and interests and their choices do not have the power to cause you to fail. It is manifested in the ability and willingness to shoulder the responsibility for meeting your own need and goals. It is manifest in the ability to be sufficiently independent of your employer, family, friends, and government to make your own determination of where your time, energy, and money will be put to use.

🌿 LOVE 🌿

Love is a special and complicated emotion which can be difficult to understand. Although most people believe that love revolves around the heart, it actually occurs in the brain. Artists, poets and painters all use the heart as the universal symbol for love, but the brain is what generates the chemical signals that make people understand love. There are different forms and styles of expressing love.

Unconditional love sees beyond the outer surface and accepts the recipient for whom they are. It is so strong that you will feel it consistently, regardless of what that other person's flaws, shortcomings or faults. It's the type of love that everyone strives to have for their fellow human beings. Although you may not like someone, you decide to love them just as a human being. This kind of love is all about sacrifice as well as giving and expecting nothing in return.

If you believe loving someone is about fostering their growth, most people acknowledge that pain and discomfort are part of growth, and if you shield someone from all pain or discomfort, you are not displaying your love properly. Do not confuse loving someone with blindly making them comfortable, satisfying their desires, and shielding them from any kind of pain. If you do, you are only making it difficult for them to grow as human beings.

Conditional love... Is it really such a thing? Can we put conditions on our love for someone? The truth is that if it's conditional, it's not love, and, sadly, much of what we call "love" isn't love at all but approval. When someone truly loves you, they love you for who you are, not for what you do. Love is as love does. It's not enough to say "I love you" if it's not followed by a loving action.

Storage love is what parents naturally feel for their children; the love that member of the family have for each other; or the love that friends feel for each other. In some cases, this friendship love may turn into a romantic relationship, and the couple in such a relationship becomes best friends. Storage love is unconditional, accepts flaws or faults and ultimately drives you to forgive. It's committed, sacrificial and makes you feel secure, comfortable and safe.

Passionate and intense love arouses your romantic feelings. It often triggers "high" feelings in a new relationship and makes you say, "I love you." It is an emotional and sexual love. Although this romantic love is important in the beginning of a new relationship, it may not last unless it moves through the three stage of love.

Lust/Erotic Passion
Lust and romantic love are two different things caused by different underlying substrates. Lust evolved for the purpose of sexual mating, while romantic love evolved because of the need for bonding, stemming from out childhood. So even though we often experience lust for our romantic partner, sometimes we don't, and that's okay. Looks and our own predispositions for what we look for in a mate play an important role in whom we lust after, as well. Without lust, we might never find that special someone. But, while lust keeps us "looking around," it is our desire for romance that leads us to attraction and love.

Romantic Passion
While the initial feelings may (or may not) come from lust, if the relationship is to progress, romantic passion must come into play. This is when we often lose our ability to think rationally. The old saying "love is blind" is really accurate in this stage. We are often oblivious to any flaws our partner might have. We idealize them and can't get them off our minds. In this stage, couples begin to spend many hours getting to know each other. If this attraction remains strong and is felt by both of them, then they usually enter the third stage: Commitment.

Commitment
This is the "love struck" phase. When you spend hours daydreaming about your loved one, you now have entered into real love. This is the period in which the bond between you and your paramour solidifies. This stage of love has to be strong enough to withstand many problems and distractions. The more we idealize the one we love, the stronger the relationship during the attachment stage.

Love is not supposed to be painful. There is pain involved in any relationship but if it is painful most of the time then you are probably in a Pathological Love Relationship because the end result of these relationships is 'Inevitable Harm.' Let's be clear that there is nothing wrong with wanting a relationship, it is natural and healthy, but we need to make sure that we are not accepting things that cause us harm for the sake of having a relationship.

What we all want and deserve is affectionate, warm and tender platonic love. This is the kind of love which livens you up. Every relationship needs love, trust and acceptance and everyone wants that something special. It takes years of love, affection and intimacy for a relationship to become strong enough for a friendship and romance to survive.

If we can start seeing relationships not as the goal but as opportunities for growth then we can start having more functional relationships. A relationship that ends is not a failure or a punishment - it is a lesson. And these lessons are mostly about pathology, its permanence, and the lives it affects without discrimination.

The truth is that there will be a million people in your life who actually don't love you, whose dismissal of your feelings or tendency to ignore what you want are rooted in genuine apathy. They are everywhere, and make

Chapter 2 | Emotional Wellness

navigating our emotional lives even more complicated. But there are also many people who do love us, and who want to show us, but just may not be able to do it in the way we most want to hear. And it's important to distinguish between the two, to look at the things people are actively doing for us and take account of the things we're lucky to have in them. Because we are lucky to have love, in any of its forms, and no way of saying "I love you" should be forgotten and said lightly.

LUST	LOVE
"Today is our 21 day anniversary"	"Has it been 5 years already?"
"How sweet, you got me flowers"	"Flowers? What did you do?"
"Good morning."	"Don't, your breathe stinks."
"She snores, it's kind of cute."	'WAKE UP! You're snoring again."
"You look so professional today."	"Are you saying I'm old? Don't answer that."
"If we had kids, they would be so adorable."	"Make sure you get the Desitin ALL the way in there."
"I love the way you smell."	"Would you please take a shower already?"

25

Emotional Wellness Assessment

Almost Always = 2 points
Sometimes/Occasionally = 1 point
Very Seldom = 0 points

____ 1. I am able to develop and maintain close relationships.
____ 2. I accept the responsibility for my actions.
____ 3. I see challenges and change as opportunities for growth.
____ 4. I feel I have considerable control over my life.
____ 5. I am able to laugh at life and myself.
____ 6. I feel good about myself.
____ 7. I am able to appropriately cope with stress and tension and make time for leisure pursuits.
____ 8. I am able to recognize my personal shortcomings and learn from my mistakes.
____ 9. I am able to recognize and express my feelings.
____ 10. I enjoy life.

_____ **Total for Emotional Wellness Dimension**

Score: **15 to 20 Points**
Excellent strength in this dimension.

Score: **9 to 14 Points**
There is room for improvement. Look again at the items in which you scored 1 or 0. What changes can you make to improve your score?

Score: **0 to 8 Points**
This dimension needs a lot of work. Look again at this dimension and challenge yourself to begin making small steps toward growth here. Remember: The goal is balanced wellness.

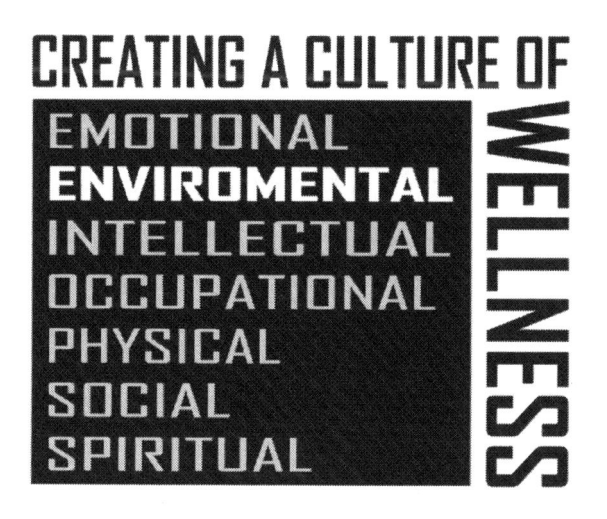

CREATING A CULTURE OF
**EMOTIONAL
ENVIROMENTAL
INTELLECTUAL
OCCUPATIONAL
PHYSICAL
SOCIAL
SPIRITUAL
WELLNESS**

Chapter 3

| Personal Impact | Social Consciousness |
| Diversity | Local Organic Food Movement |
| Sustainable Development |

Environmental Wellness for an adult encompasses acknowledging the interdependence between man and the earth and other living beings. Maintaining and replenishing the resources we need to support current and future life is the goal. Caring for the animals and places that are entrusted to you in a way that ensures continued viability for all life forms demonstrates environmental maturity. Designing work and play spaces that enable full healthful function while maximizing usability is desirable. Cultivating an appreciation for the beauty found in nature and surrounding yourself with rejuvenating, comforting, and affirming places and people contributes to your ability to refresh and revitalize yourself and enhance full capacity wellness capabilities.

🌿 PERSONAL IMPACT 🌿

Environmental personal impact is also known as ones "Carbon Footprint." Carbon footprints measure how much carbon dioxide (CO_2) we produce just by going about our daily lives. A drive to work, a flip of a light switch and a flight out of town all rely on the combustion of fossil fuels like oil, coal and gas. When fossil fuels burn, they emit greenhouse gases like CO_2 that contribute to global warming.

Each day, you make dozens of energy-related decisions. Some of these decisions are based on comfort and convenience, and others may take into account the impact in your gas or electric bill. When making choices about appliance use, it is important to know how much it costs to operate a certain appliance, not only in dollars but in environmental impact.

People concerned with the environment and global warming usually try to reduce their carbon output by increasing their home's energy efficiency and driving less. Some start by calculating their carbon footprint to set a benchmark, like a weigh-in before a diet. A carbon footprint is simply a figure, usually a monthly or annual total of CO_2 output measured in tons. Web sites with carbon footprint calculators turn information like annual mileage and monthly power usage into a measurable number for you. Most people try to reduce their carbon footprint, but others aim to erase it completely.

When people attempt carbon neutrality, they cut their emissions as much as possible and offset the rest. Carbon offsets let you pay to reduce the global greenhouse gas total instead of making radical reductions of your own. When you buy an offset, you fund projects that reduce emissions by restoring forests, updating power plants and factories or increasing the energy efficiency of buildings and transportation.

The amount of municipal solid waste (household and commercial waste) that the average person generates varies widely by country. According to the World Resources Institute, some typical waste generation rates are:

United States:	4.4lbs/person/day
Canada:	3.9bs/person/day
Spain:	1.7lbs/person/day
Finland:	1.5lbs/person/day

The environmental impact of this consumption varies with how much recycling and composting is done in your region. The primary impacts are natural resource use, energy use, and the air emissions associated with energy use.

Individual water use is really a drop in the bucket. While per capita water use is about 1400 gallons per day in the U.S., the amount used directly by an individual is only a small part of that.

Agriculture:	41%
Electric Generation Cooling:	38%
Industry:	11%
Public Tab Water:	10%

There are many regional differences in the amount of water used. In the West, most of the water is used for irrigation, while in the East more water is used by industry. Residential water use is affected not only by water conservation equipment, like low flow showerheads, but by personal actions, like the amount of time you spend in the shower.

How you get around can have a big impact on the environment. Cars, trucks, and other passenger vehicles spew out 20 percent of U.S. carbon dioxide (CO_2) emissions. CO_2 is a major contributor to global warming. These vehicles also account for about half of U.S. oil consumption. Thus every driver is somewhat responsible for the millions of gallons of oil that get spilled every year. Passenger vehicles are the largest sources of carbon monoxide (a poisonous gas). They are also major producers of hydrocarbon emissions (which help form ground level ozone, "smog") and nitrogen oxides (which help form smog and acid rain).

🌱 Social Consciousness 🌱

Simply put the recognition and realization that we are all connected. We are connected in ways that we may not even realize, but if you accept that fact, you will start to look at everything you encounter and every person you interact with as a part of you, you are being socially conscious. Being socially conscious means that essentially you are following the Golden Rule at all times with people, business, nature and most importantly your thoughts. We want humans to be more humane and work cooperatively as a unit rather than as separated pieces. Having read this you have already changed and are becoming more awake and conscious whether you realize it or not.

In Level One of social consciousness is what we refer to as embedded. Here consciousness is shaped without our awareness by social, cultural, and biological factors. It's a kind of pre-social consciousness that serves as a baseline for our own development. Social factors interact with our cognitive and biological processes, limiting our ability to know what shapes our inner experiences. We see what we expect to see – and can consistently miss things we are not anticipating or that don't support our belief system.

With greater human choice and creativity, we may begin to express our human spirit in the face of on-going social and political influences. This leads to Level Two, which we call self-reflexive social consciousness. Here people gain awareness of how their experiences are conditioned by the social world. This can be accomplished through personal reflection and contemplative practices such as meditation. Scientists and spiritual teachers alike are working together to broaden our awareness of the world and our place in it.

Psychologist and religious historian Louise Sundararajan emphasizes that it is the capacity for self-reflexivity, the ability to step back and reflect on our thought process, which stimulate shifts in our mental representations. From insight meditation to the confessional in the Catholic tradition, to taking inventory of one's behavior in the 12 step programs, each practice can help us to become more self-aware. In this process, we can begin to analyze our own biases and remove our perceptual blinders.

Level Three is what we term engaged social consciousness. At this stage, we are not only aware of the social environment but begin to mobilize our intention to contribute to the greater good. There is a movement from "me" to "we" as our awareness moves us to actively engage in the well-being of others and the world. There is also an expansion of perspective-taking, in which we get better at seeing things from another person's point of view. Scientific data from interpersonal neurobiology suggests that our brains develop through our connections to others. Additional data points to build in drives within us that lead us to search for purpose in our lives, suggesting that our brains are social organs.

Level Four involves what we call collaborative social consciousness. Gaining greater awareness of ourselves in relation to the social world may lead us to participate in co-creating solutions with others. Here we begin to shape the social environment through collaborative actions. Within education, for example, we find an increasing focus on participatory learning, service learning, and project-based learning. Each was developed to enhance the nature of collaborative social consciousness through discourse and conversation. Wisdom Cafes, Open Space Technology, and Bohemian Dialogue Groups offer collaborative explorations and life-affirming actions.

Level Five is what we call resonant consciousness. At this stage of development people, report a sense of essential interrelatedness with others. They describe a "field" of shared experience and emergence that is felt and expressed in social groups. Mystical states of interconnectedness, deep rapport, unspoken communication, have all been expressed by spiritual teachers, educators, and psychologists alike, as a stage in social consciousness. These notions are further developed by research, such as that conducted at ions, that speak to measurable links between one person's intention and another person's physiological activity, revealing an underlying entanglement between us. Such studies are evocative and provide an empirical basis for connections that lie beyond our physical relations.

🌾 DIVERSITY 🌾

The United States is becoming increasingly diverse. By the turn of the century one out of every three Americans will be a person of color. According to James Banks, more than 8 million legal immigrants came to the U.S. between 1981 and 1990, and an undetermined number of undocumented immigrants enter the United States each year. In addition, the United States includes people of many religions, languages, economic groups, and other cultural groups.

Culture is a strong part of people's lives. It influences their views, their values, their humor, their hopes, their loyalties, and their worries and fears. If you are from New Mexico or Montana, if your parents are Cambodian, French Canadian, or Native American, if you are German Catholic or African-American, if you are Jewish or Mormon, if you are straight or Gay, if you are a mixture of cultures your culture has affected you. So when you are working with people and building relationships with them, it helps to have some perspective and understanding of their cultures.

But as we explore culture, it's also important to remember how much we have in common. A person who grew up in Tibet, will probably see the world very differently than someone who grew up in Manhattan, but both people know what it is like to wake up in the morning and look forward to the adventures that of the day. We are all human beings. We all love deeply, want to learn, have hopes and dreams, and have experienced pain and fear.

At the same time, we can't pretend that our cultures and differences don't matter. We can't gloss over differences and pretend they don't exist, wishing that we could be alike. We cannot pretend that discrimination doesn't exist.

People have very different views of what a multicultural society or community should be like or could be like. In the past few decades there has been a lot of discussion about what it means to live and work together in a society that is diverse as ours. People struggle with different visions of a fair, equitable, moral, and harmonious society.

LOCAL ORGANIC FOOD MOVEMENT

Most people are aware of the health risks associated with chemicals, such as, pesticides, asbestos, carbon monoxide and other toxic chemicals. The organic food movement reflects several overlapping themes about healthful food and environmental sustainability. The big questions is, do you know where you food comes from?

In our current food system shipping food long distances for processing and packaging, importing and exporting foods that don't need to be imported or exported, these are standard practices in the food industry. Simply put, if you drive a mile away from a large farm and sit in a café, the food on your table most likely have traveled about 1, 500 miles before arriving on your plate. This is due to the food being grown at one location, processed at another, and then package yet at another location. These locations frequently are located all over the county, not close to the actual food producer.

How fresh can that really be? What additives had to be added to that tomato sauce to ensure it could make the trip back to your table without going bad? These are the questions you should be asking. The next time you are at the grocery store or supermarket look at the label to see where your food comes from. I guarantee you will be shocked.

Films such as Food, Inc., Fresh, King Corn, Genetic Roulette, and The Future of Food have done just that and exposed many to the fact that much of what is available in the seemingly unprecedented selection of the supermarket are really just reconfigurations of corn and soy, or things that were fed using corn and soy. These foods typically won't rot, while you can eat it, but should you. The United States is started to see an awakening of food consciousness in the general public that wasn't there a decade ago. This is making the voice of small, local-based farmers heard, and their voice is getting louder.

Public concern is growing over the long-term safety of genetically altered food, hormones, antibiotics, pesticides, the health of the soil, toxic chemicals in the water, humane treatment of farm animals, and even the health of those essential pollinators, bees. As the concern grows, so does support for local farmers who choose to grow organic.

The Local Organic Food Movement, which advocates local, clean, non-adulterated, sustainable food, is making its way back into our society. Local small producing farms are growing and selling good quality, intensely tasteful, sustainable, organic, clean food for local populations of people. We are starting to see the reemergence of communities being formed around local food production.

There are thousands of locally owned farms that are committed to staying reasonably-sized, feeding people locally, and assisting others into local food production such as small community gardens, container gardens, and recently hydroponic and aquaponic gardening.

Farmers who know their land, crops, and animals intimately can take better care of them and elating the need for millions of tons of antibiotics, pesticides, and other toxic chemicals in and on the food we eat. The idea of small farms allows us to see the productiveness of farming in terms of personal and environmental health rather than merely as a business.

The tide is turning in favor of local, healthy produced food, and people are staring in the face of a very anemic economy. The roots of America are in the soil, and the original vision of America's founding fathers was highly agrarian. With the right support, a few small to medium-sized farms could make a dramatic difference in one's local community.

SUSTAINABLE DEVELOPMENT

The term "sustainable development" has several definitions. A common denominator is that living standards for human beings must improve, but without jeopardizing the possibility for future generations to enjoy equally good conditions. We live in a highly dynamic, human-dominated earth system in which non-linear, abrupt and irreversible changes are not only possible but also probable

Much people in this world are vulnerable to natural disasters, extreme poverty, infectious disease and a host of other challenges. One in six people on the planet live off of less than $1 a day. The world's population is expected to increase to nine billion by 2050. Human activity is straining the planet's resources, threatening the health of our environment and ability to thrive. Balancing human demand for land and food with the need to protect the world's dwindling natural resources is a global challenge.

Unsustainable development has increased the stress on the earth's limited natural resources, and on the carrying capacity of ecosystem, and will continue to do so until all of us do something about it. For developing nations, the challenge can seem insurmountable in the face of booming populations, entrenched poverty and limited institutional know-how for creating sustainable resource management policies. Developing nations can also miss out on tapping into the vast economic benefits that can come with reducing environmental damage and over-exploitation.

In recent years, sustainable building practices have become much more prominent among homebuilders, architects, developers, and city planners in the construction of residential and commercial buildings and communities. Sustainable development includes creation of homes, buildings, and businesses that meet the needs of the people who occupy them, while enhancing human and environmental health.

Sustainable development can be achieved through multiple initiatives that a community or individual can do. Here are a few areas of interest that you must think about when trying to improve sustainability.

Water

Climate variability and change are making it difficult to provide water where and when it is needed. Floods destroy communities in one part of the world, while in another people walk miles every day just to get enough water to survive.

Energy

Carbon dioxide is altering Earth's climate. Fossil fuels are abundant and relatively cheap but emit large amounts of carbon dioxide, we must find ways to make the burning of fossil fuels less polluting. In order to reduce the effects of global climate change while still allowing for continued economic development, we need to develop alternative energy sources and increase energy efficiency

Urbanization

Urban areas provide economic opportunity, the potential for increased efficiency and improvements in standard of living, but they are also under acute stress as their populations expand. This in turn puts pressure on the areas that support their resource needs, creating social, infrastructural and health challenges to the sustainability of cities.

When you think of the world as a system over space, you grow to understand that air pollution from North America affects air quality in Asia, and that pesticides sprayed in Argentina could harm fish stocks off the coast of Australia. When you begin to think of the world as an interrelated, over time you will start to realize that the decisions our grandparents made about how to farm the land continue to affect agricultural practice today, and the policies we put into place today will have an impact on our children are adults.

People concerned about sustainable development suggest that meeting the needs of the future depends on how well we balance social, economic, and environmental needs, or needs, when making decisions today. Many of these needs may seem to conflict with each other in the short term. For example, industrial growth might conflict with preserving natural resources. Yet, in the long term, responsible use of natural resources now will help ensure that there are resources available for sustained industrial growth far into the future.

The way we approach development affects everyone. The impacts of our decisions as a society have very real consequences for people's lives. Poor planning of communities, for example, reduces the quality of life for the people who live in them. Sustainable development provides an approach to making better decisions on the issues that affect all of our lives.

Environmental Wellness Assessment

Almost always = 2 points
Sometimes/occasionally = 1 point
Very seldom = 0 points

____ 1. I consciously conserve energy (electricity, heat, light, water, etc.) in my place of residence.
____ 2. I practice recycling (glass, paper, plastic, etc.)
____ 3. I am committed to cleaning up the environment (air, soil, water, etc.)
____ 4. I consciously try to conserve fuel energy and to lessen the pollution in the atmosphere.
____ 5. I limit the use of fertilizers and chemicals when managing my yard/lawn/outdoor living space.
____ 6. I do not use aerosol sprays.
____ 7. I do not litter.
____ 8. I volunteer my time for environmental conservation projects.
____ 9. I purchase recycled items when possible, even if they cost more.
____ 10. I feel very strongly about doing my part to preserve the environment.

____ **Total for Environmental Wellness Dimension**

Score: **15 to 20 Points**
Excellent strength in this dimension.

Score: **9 to 14 Points**
There is room for improvement. Look again at the items in which you scored 1 or 0. What changes can you make to improve your score?

Score: **0 to 8 Points**
This dimension needs a lot of work. Look again at this dimension and challenge yourself to begin making small steps toward growth here. Remember: The goal is balanced wellness.

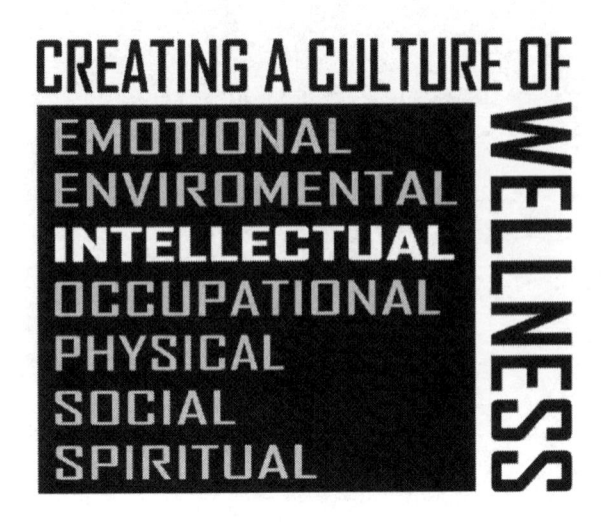

CREATING A CULTURE OF
EMOTIONAL
ENVIROMENTAL
INTELLECTUAL
OCCUPATIONAL
PHYSICAL
SOCIAL
SPIRITUAL
WELLNESS

Chapter 4

| Problem Solving | Education | Knowledge |
| Personal Growth | Decision Making |

Intellectual wellness for adults involves embracing lifetime learning. The realization that learning doesn't end once you have completed a formal education is key to growing and changing in order to continually respond to the world around us. Maintaining a sense of wonder and curiosity and staying intellectually stimulated helps sustain a vital existence long into the lifespan. There is a constant human need and desire to be creative and innovative, and a need to constantly need to explore new and exciting subjects while expanding our knowledge of our environment and of the unknown. Finding a way to express these qualities is life affirming. Using knowledge effectively in all aspects in your life, with friends or family, in work or volunteer efforts is a never ending process. An intellectually mature person seeks to discover and understand many divergent points of view, even if they conflict, in order to develop an informed personal point of view. Acquiring new skills, developing new ideas, having the ability to interpret and articulate what you think about what you've learned contributes to being intellectually well.

🎋 Problem Solving 🎋

We continuously bump up against obstacles that stand between us and what we need or want. For the most part, we are able to quickly solve them without much trouble at all. We either come up with a quick solution or use a strategy that worked in the past. Everybody can benefit from having good problem solving skills. It would be beneficial to have the ability to solve all problems efficiently and in a timely fashion without difficulty, unfortunately there is no one way in which all problems can be solved.

Problem-solving can mean the world in a place of differences. Finding common ground without being afraid to disagree is key to improving any relationship, personal or professionally. It will assist in getting things done democratically and effectively. There are some benefits to successful problem solving:

- ❖ Building better solutions
- ❖ Dealing with more stakeholders
- ❖ Completing more complex tasks
- ❖ Learn to make new mistakes, not the same old ones.

There are a couple of different ways to problem solve, and some handy tips and tricks you can use. If the below action steps don't work, there are a number of other things you can try to see what works best for you.

Define the Problem
What prevents you from reaching your goal? State the problem in broad terms since the exact problem may not be obvious. You may lack information to define it or you can confuse symptoms with underlying causes. Prepare a statement of the problem and find someone you trust to talk it over with. If the problem is a job situation, review it with your supervisor or the appropriate committee or resource.

Develop and Weigh Alternatives
Look at your problems in different ways and try to find a new perspective that you haven't thought of before. Brainstorming or rapid note taking, or use of any other alternatives no matter how silly may be the key as well. Once you have listed or mapped alternatives, be open to all the possibilities.

Implement Decision
Develop a plan for implementation, a step-by-step process or actions. Then create strong communication strategy for notifying other key stakeholders. Where important or necessary, inform those who care for you and/or will be affected by the change. Identify the resources needed and create a timeline for implementation. Your implementation will only be successful if you are monitoring your solution, the effects of it on resources, others it has involved, your timeline, and progress. As you monitor your progress, if results are not what you expect, review your options and alternatives.

Experience both lets us know the constraints to a problem, as well as what steps we must take in solving the problem. More specifically, when solving a problem, we are using our experience to tell us which changes we must make to get from our initial state to the final state. Solving problems in which you do not have all the specific experience to propose a solution is risky. Even after applying the experience of others, making estimates, or making assumptions, it may turn out that your proposed solution doesn't work. Even though you must go back and propose a different solution to the problem, this is not always a bad thing, because now you have experience for the next time you encounter the same, or similar, problem. You now know in what cases a proposed solution absolutely won't work, which cases might work, and which cases appear to always solve the problem.

EDUCATION

In today's world, a good education is essential. Not only will one be able to make better decisions in life, but also obtain higher pay and respectable careers with a good education. Education is not all about studying and getting good marks. It is really a means to discover new things that we don't know about and increase our knowledge. An educated person has the ability to differentiate between right and wrong or good and evil. It is the foremost responsibility of a society to educate its citizens.

A good education not only teaches one the essential skills of the working world; it also prepares the mind to make sane, healthy, and intelligent decisions about any situation that one may encounter in life's journey. A good education helps one to determine between what is right and what is wrong. Although there are several benefits to a good education, the main benefit is that it makes one a better person in all aspects of life. A person becomes perfect with education as he is not only gaining something from it, but also contributing to the growth of a nation.

Back in the 30's and 40's, only a small proportion of Americans went to college. They didn't need to. Most jobs didn't require degrees. Everything has changed. People who don't get some kind of post-secondary education are quickly falling out of the American middle class. Today, nearly 60% of all jobs in the U.S. economy require higher education. The wage gap between people who have bachelor's degrees and people with a high school diploma has nearly doubled since the early 1980s.

College-educated people not only tend to have higher earnings than people without degrees, they are also more likely to have health and retirement benefits with their jobs, and they are far less likely to be unemployed. Having a degree is not just about economic advantages; people with college degrees are more likely to be satisfied with their jobs. They are more likely to read to their children, which helps their kids be better prepared for school than other children.

Despite the fact that enrollment in college has increased in the last ten years the high school dropout rate is still a serious issue in the United States. Each year, over 1.2 million American students drop out of high school. Many of today's high school dropouts are struggling to make ends meet. Over a lifetime, students who are unable to finish high school earn an average of $200,000 less than their peers who graduate from high school and $800,000 less than their peers who graduate from college. Students who are unable to complete high school comprise about half of the heads of households on welfare, and many of these households are headed by women who were teenage parents.

High school dropout rates are a serious nationwide issue. It not only impacts the millions of students who drop out of school but it affects the economic stability of the nation at large. Communities have to be dedicated to education and have advocates on the side of all at-risk youth to ensure that they have equal access and equal quality education. Everyone can play a role in reducing the high school dropout rate by tutoring students in local high schools, volunteering with dropout prevention programs, and mentoring young people.

We can say that education is simply the soul of a society, as it passes from one generation to another. It is also is universally recognized as one of the most fundamental building blocks for human development and poverty reduction. When given the opportunity to learn, people are empowered to contribute fully to the development of their lives, their communities, and their countries. Education remains one of the most powerful instruments for reducing poverty and inequality, and helps lay the foundation for sustained economic growth.

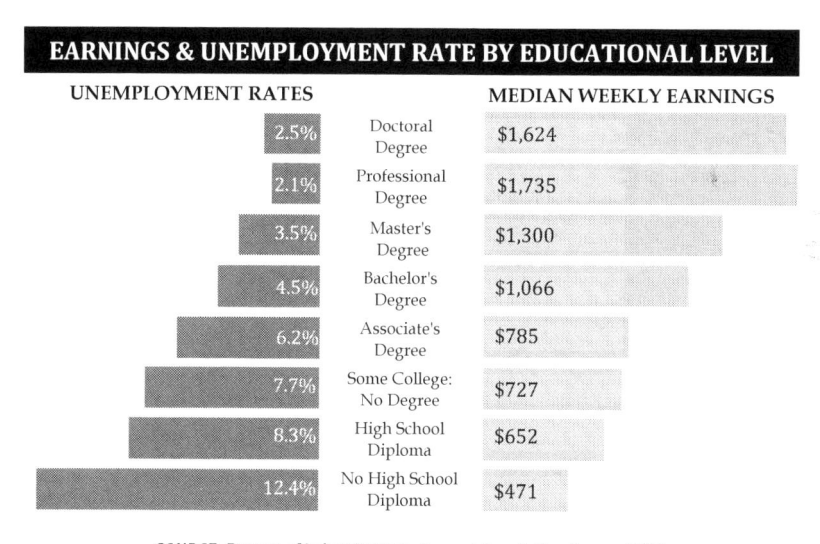

EARNINGS & UNEMPLOYMENT RATE BY EDUCATIONAL LEVEL

UNEMPLOYMENT RATES		MEDIAN WEEKLY EARNINGS
2.5%	Doctoral Degree	$1,624
2.1%	Professional Degree	$1,735
3.5%	Master's Degree	$1,300
4.5%	Bachelor's Degree	$1,066
6.2%	Associate's Degree	$785
7.7%	Some College: No Degree	$727
8.3%	High School Diploma	$652
12.4%	No High School Diploma	$471

SOURCE: Bureau of Labor Staticits, Current Pupolation Surve - 2012

🦋 KNOWLEDGE 🦋

Knowledge, in effect, is the accumulation of facts, myths, trivia and beliefs. It's an all-encompassing field of data that we use to live by from methods to complete a task, data to be able to plan as well as the ability to reflect on what was learned. By and large, the amount of knowledge we have is far greater than the amount of it we really understand.

Knowledge, when closely observed, reveals itself to be entirely linked to the past, but not the present moment. All our knowledge and information has been accumulated over a long period of time, the present moment simply is - there is just awareness and being. It is important to consider this aspect.

It has long said that the principal method of gaining knowledge is through the five senses. Socrates, a great ancient Greek philosopher, believed differently. He thought that we will never learn the reality and truth of anything if we continue to rely on our senses. No two people will ever hear or see the same thing in an identical way and consequently, will never process the information in the same way either. The complication arises now, is understanding and knowledge the same thing? Is knowledge different for everyone?

Most people go through life with no understanding of what they're doing or what they actually know. In your life you will gain large amounts of knowledge with hopes that that they will magically be understood. After years go by, more knowledge is gained and eventually you begin to lose track of the fact that you don't understand most of it. Or at best, you understand it only in a minimal, completely self-referential, manner. Knowledge and understanding are fundamentally different.

Perhaps the "secret ingredient" of all knowledge is the ability to understand, having the insight to where not only the concept is understood, but its practical application makes perfect sense as well. By and large, the amount of knowledge you have is far greater than the amount of it you really understand. There is very little knowledge that you haven't come across through education, experiences, or from personal study, but the retention of data is simply the retention of data that is not obtained "now." The data that was obtained "then" and is now stored for personal use in our minds is our understanding of the past as use it as knowledge for the future. The greater deal of understanding happens when the knowledge previously learned is applied.

The gaining of knowledge and understanding is a journey. Even if we end up in the same location in the physical sense, it is our duty to take the journey, and use it to gain a deeper insight into ourselves and the world around us. Maybe, in the present moment there is simply understanding, which may lead to knowledge in the future.

🌿 Personal Growth 🌿

Personal growth and development is a transformational process, in which improvements are made in your physical, emotional, intellectual, spiritual, social, and/or financial state. This process is often triggered by an important life event that inspires you to improve and empower yourself by discovering where your full potential lies. The result is a more satisfying and meaningful life, which is evident in your relationships, place of work, self-image and self-confidence, as well as your world view.

Once this process is underway the results are endless. You will find meaning and purpose in yourself that was absent before. Life goals will become possible. You will use your full potential to benefit yourself and others. New skills and talents will be discovered. Old relationships will be strengthened and new ones will be easily formed. All of which will give you a boost in your self-image and self-confidence. Every person is a unique individual and because of this, a universal strategy for personal growth and development cannot exist. Each pathway towards personal growth and development is a personalized journey. It is up to the individual to figure out which pathway is theirs and where it leads.

Perhaps the most difficult part of changing your life involves exploring your inner world. True change cannot just occur on the surface or outside of you. Change means not only understanding who you are, but also why you are who you are, in other words, what makes you tick. The first step you must take is to identify the obstacles that are preventing you from changing. You need to "look in the mirror" and specify what the baggage, habits, emotions, and environment are keeping you from your goals. Understanding these obstacles takes the mystery out of who you are and what has been holding you back. It also gives you clarity on what you need to change and gives you an initial direction in your path of change.

These explorations of your inner world can enable you to finally understand why you have been the way you have been and done things you have done even when neither have worked for you. This process will also help you to remove the obstacles that have stood in your path to change. These insights also, at a deep level, liberate you to move from your current path to another that will take you where you really want to go. Most importantly, truly understanding your inner world will allow you to finally put the past behind you-when most of your life you have been putting your past in front of you.

If we are interested in personal growth, no element is more important than developing a love of truth. Seeking the truth means being curious about what is going on in ourselves and around us, not settling for the automatic answers our personality feeds us. If we observe ourselves, we will see that many of the stock explanations that we give ourselves for our behavior or for the actions of others are a form of resistance. As we learn to accept what is real in the present moment, we are more able to accept whatever arises in us, because we know that it is not the whole of us. The truth encompasses both our fearful reactions and the greater resources of our soul. While our automatic reactions can derail our search for the truth, acknowledging their presence brings us closer to the truth. When we are willing to be with the whole truth, whatever it is, we have more inner resources available to deal with whatever we are facing.

Decision Making

Decision-making is a key skill in the workplace, and is particularly important if you want to be an effective leader. Whether you're deciding which person to hire, which supplier to use, or which strategy to pursue, the ability to make a good decision with available information is vital. It would be easy if there were one formula you could use in any situation, but there isn't. Each decision presents its own challenges, and we all have different ways of approaching problems. Decision making is an essential leadership skill. If you can learn how to make timely, well-considered decisions, then you can lead your team to well-deserved success.

Making decisions that produce successful results for your department or organization makes you look good and makes you promotable for leadership. Supervisors appreciate employees who are good decision makers because it allows them the freedom to focus on coaching and other aspects of their jobs. Poor decision making does not bode well for your career in many instances. Some jobs with minimal decision making exist, but moving up and making more money are usually not as easy if you make poor decisions. Limited upward mobility is not the only drawback of bad decisions. You may also alienate or upset colleagues or team members with constant mistakes that affect them. Even more extreme, you could lose your job if your decisions have very negative consequences for your company.

So, how do you avoid making bad decisions, or leaving decisions to chance? You need a systematic approach to decision-making so that, no matter what type of decision you have to make, you can take decisions with confidence. No one can afford to make poor decisions. If, however, you make poor decisions, your time as a leader will be brutally short.

If you've ever been in a meeting where people seem to be discussing different issues, then you've seen what happens when the decision-making environment hasn't been established. It's so important for everyone to understand the issue before preparing to make a decision. This includes agreeing on an objective, making sure the right issue is being discussed, and agreeing on a process to move the decision forward. You also must address key interpersonal considerations at the very beginning. Have you included all the stakeholders? And do the people involved in the decision agree to respect one another and engage in an open and honest discussion? After all, if only the strongest opinions are heard, you risk not considering some of the best solutions available.

Another important part of a good decision making process is generating as many good alternatives as possible to consider. If you simply adopt the first solution you encounter, then you're probably missing a number of better alternatives. Remember that some things about a decision are not objective. The decision has to make sense on an intuitive, instinctive level as well. The entire process we have discussed so far has been based on the perspectives and experiences of all the people involved. Now it's time to check the alternative you've chosen for validity and "making sense." If the decision is a significant one, it's also worth auditing it to make sure that your assumptions are correct, and that the logical structure you've used to make the decision is sound.

You can try to force your decision on others by demanding their acceptance. Or you can gain their acceptance by explaining how and why you reached your decision. For most decisions, particularly those that need participant buy-in before implementation, it's more effective to gather support by explaining your decision. Have a plan for implementing your decision. People usually respond positively to a clear plan, one that tells them what to expect and what they need to do.

Ultimately, it is your job to make decisions that are in the best interest for you and of the organization. You must consider the good of many, not of a few. This is a big responsibility and very often people don't appreciate your efforts. Take a moment and learn about different decision making styles, one may not be suitable for all decisions so you must be familiar with multiple styles.

Democratic

Democratic decision making is when the leader gives up ownership and control of a decision and allows the group to vote. Majority vote will decide the action. Advantages include a fairly fast decision, and a certain amount of group participation. The disadvantage of this style includes no responsibility.

Autocratic

Autocratic decision making is when you are the one who maintains total control and ownership of the decision. You are also completely responsible for the good or bad outcome as a result of the decision. You do not ask for any suggestions or ideas from outside sources and you decide on your own information and perception of the situation. Advantages include a very fast decision, and personal responsibility by the leader, for the outcome. The disadvantages are varied and sometimes include less than desired effort from the people that must carry it out.

Collective
Collective decision making is when you involve all the members of the organization. Gathering and involving other's ideas, perceptions, knowledge, and information concerning the decision. Advantages include some group participation and involvement. The disadvantages of this style include a fairly slow, time consuming decision; less security, because so many people are involved in the decision.

Consensus
Consensus decision making is when you give up total control of the decision. The complete group is totally involved in the decision. The complete organization or group is now responsible for the outcome. This is not a democratic style because *everyone* must agree and "buy in" on the decision. If total commitment and agreement by everyone is not obtained the decision becomes democratic. Advantages include group commitment and responsibility for the outcome. The disadvantages include a very slow and extremely time consuming decision. It is also a lot of work getting everyone in the organization involved.

INTELLECTUAL WELLNESS ASSESSMENT

Almost Always = 2 points
Sometimes/Occasionally = 1 point
Very Seldom = 0 points

____ 1. I am interested in learning new things.
____ 2. I try to keep abreast of current affairs - locally, nationally, and internationally.
____ 3. I enjoy attending lectures, plays, musical performances, museums, galleries, and/or libraries.
____ 4. I carefully select movies and television programs.
____ 5. I enjoy creative and stimulating mental activities/games.
____ 6. I am happy with the amount and variety that I read.
____ 7. I make an effort to improve my verbal and written skills.
____ 8. A continuing education program is/will be important to me in my career.
____ 9. I am able to analyze, synthesize, and see more than one side of an issue.
____ 10. I enjoy engaging in intellectual discussions.

____ Total for Intellectual Wellness Dimension

Score: **15 to 20 Points**
Excellent strength in this dimension.

Score: **9 to 14 Points**
There is room for improvement. Look again at the items in which you scored 1 or 0. What changes can you make to improve your score?

Score: **0 to 8 Points**
This dimension needs a lot of work. Look again at this dimension and challenge yourself to begin making small steps toward growth here. Remember: The goal is balanced wellness.

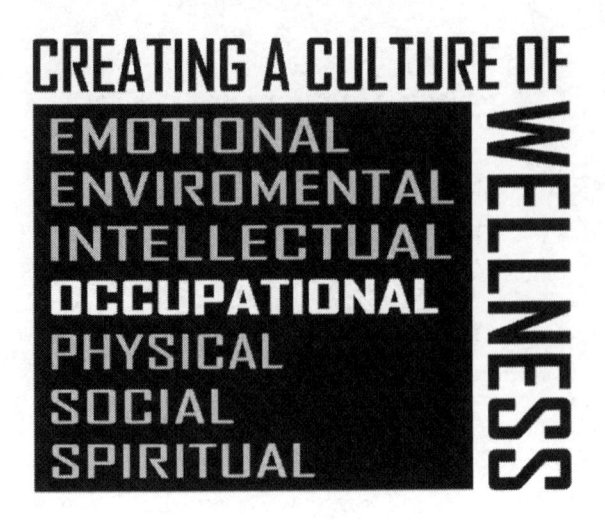

CREATING A CULTURE OF
EMOTIONAL
ENVIROMENTAL
INTELLECTUAL
OCCUPATIONAL
PHYSICAL
SOCIAL
SPIRITUAL
WELLNESS

Chapter 5

| Job Satisfaction | Career Opportunity |
| Job Skills | Position | Career Goals |
| Healthy Working Environment |

    Hating your job, overworking yourself, and feeling like you aren't living to your full potential are signs that your occupational wellness is suffering. In order to have good occupational wellness, you need to balance work and leisure. Finding satisfaction in your career is also important, as well as feeling comfortable and valued at your place of work.

    Wellness for adults includes being able to identify your skills, abilities, and interests in order to incorporate them into your life's work. Being willing to continually learn and explore many career options keeps you flexible and able to respond to different economic cycles. Becoming a lifelong learner opens new possibilities for finding talents, interests, and passions that may develop into a career. Working at a job that you feel passionate about enables you to obtain a higher job satisfaction. Putting your skills and abilities to use, you gain a sense of purpose and meaning and enrich your life. A vocationally mature person seeks to find a healthy balance between social and work life and has examined many different interpretations of success to define what it may mean for him or herself. An educated person sets goals and outlines ways to attain them.

JOB SATISFACTION

The American workplace can be very unforgiving. It tends to demand longer hours and offer fewer benefits and vacation time than its counterparts in other areas of the world. It's a little bit of a revelation, then, to discover that people in this country actually have a relatively high rate of satisfaction in their jobs.

Job satisfaction provides a broad measure of how content American workers are in their jobs. American workers generally say they are satisfied with their work, though slightly fewer than in 2008. It is unclear the cause of the decline in job satisfaction, though in recent years there have been reports of employees taking on more and less-than-ideal work as companies reduced staff and of workers having to take jobs they are overqualified for after losing their previous job. Concerns about job security, heightened by high unemployment, are likely playing a role as well.

If you've gone sour on your job, take some time to think about what motivates and inspires you — and how you approach your work. Basically there are three ways to look at your job.

It's just a job
If you approach work as a job, you focus primarily on the financial rewards. The nature of the work may hold little interest for you. What's important is the money. If a job with more pay comes your way, you'll move on.

It's a career
If you approach work as a career, you're likely interested in advancement. Your current job may just be a steppingstone to your ultimate goal. What's important is to be regarded as a success in your field.

This is my calling
If you approach your job as a calling, you focus on the work itself. You're less interested in financial gain or career advancement, preferring instead to find a sense of fulfillment from the work itself.

One approach isn't necessarily better, and you might find elements of all three perspectives important. Still, if you're unsatisfied with your job, it's helpful to reflect on why you work. Think about what originally drew you to your current job, and whether it may be a factor in your lack of job satisfaction. Understanding what motivates you in your work can help you reframe your expectations and make choices to increase your satisfaction.

Career Opportunity

The recession of 2007-2009, millions of Americans are still out of work, and the recovery is largely meaningless. All Americans saw significant job losses during this recession and comparatively high unemployment rates persist for all. In addition, because poor economic conditions are an important causal factor behind poor educational outcomes and high crime rates are correlated with high unemployment rates, creating job opportunities would help improve educational outcomes and reduce crime.

"There is no scarcity of opportunity to make a living at what you love; there's only scarcity of resolve to make it happen."
- Wayne Dyer -

    If you want to change roles or get ahead in your career, it's important that you know how to identify and pursue opportunities that are a good match for your interests, skills, and circumstances. This takes time. You can think of the process of finding opportunities as a journey that will eventually lead you to an exciting but unknown destination. You need to be patient, and persist in your efforts. That being said, work that you put in now will pay off in the future. Not only will you end up in a role that's right for you, but you'll have a good understanding of your options. What's more, people will think of you when new openings come up, and you won't waste time pursuing the wrong opportunities. You'll also have a better understanding of where you need to build new skills, and develop existing ones to be successful in your career.

    Most people will agree that when it comes to career advancement, the ladder to success can be a steep one to climb. One of the ways to improve your career advancement opportunities and be a step ahead of your rivals is to work harder and do some serious planning and preparation. Here are some things that may help you in your career development:

Have the Right Mindset
Opportunities are all around you, all of the time. So you need to be continually watching out for them. Get into the habit of looking for possible opportunities every day. Keep a notebook with you, or use a smartphone app like 'Evernote' to keep track of new opportunities when you think of them. Write down as many possible opportunities as you can, you can trim your list back to the most relevant opportunities later on.

Be Flexible
In a scenario of political flip-flops and economic uncertainty, professionals need to be extremely flexible. "For leaders, it is about building a structure, which responds to the market scenario quickly when new policies are announced. As individuals, you need to be ready to lap up the next big break.

Seek Opportunities
You will need to make an effort to seek out "hidden" opportunities. These are opportunities like job openings that aren't advertised, and projects that you can initiate because you have spotted an unfulfilled need within your organization or industry. Make sure that you stay up-to-date on your industry, so that you're aware of relevant trends and new technologies, these often create. Begin with your organization. Keep an eye on current internal or upcoming vacancies, and on any plans for the organization to expand. Also, think about how you could progress in the organization from your current position - what paths are available to you?

Choose a Mentor

A career mentor can be very beneficial to your future success. A mentor is an experienced business person who has already navigated to the top of your chosen career and will show you how to do the same. But success is not the only qualification for a good mentor. A mentor must have a strong desire to share his or her accumulated wisdom and to give something back to the professional community. Finding the right business mentor is a long process, and it should be. Think of it like dating. You shouldn't settle for the first silver-haired, six-figure executive that comes along. Try to find an experienced and trustworthy individual who has both the time and inclination to invest in your future success.

JOB SKILLS

If you think you don't have any experience, you may want to think about that again! You may not have specific job experience, but you do have work experience. With competition for new jobs at an all-time high, employees must have the skills employers are targeting. Creating a job skills development plan is a useful strategy for achieving professional growth. The ideal plan identifies long-term goals and outlines a detailed approach for developing job skills. It is the idea that the skills of U.S. workers don't match the needs of the nation's employers.

This "job skills mismatch" is routinely the reason why most believe why the unemployment rate is still high after the 2007-2008 recessions, and why nearly half of those out of work have been so for more than six months. When companies are asked why they have difficulty hiring, 55% say that the there is a lack of available applicants. The conversation revolves around whether workers have the right skills for the jobs they are applying for or not. If they do have the right job skills for the position, are companies willing to pay enough to compensate workers for having acquired those skills? When firms post job openings at a certain wage and no one comes forward, we call this a skills mismatch.

The skills mismatch is a simple tale to tell. There is a thing called a worker and a thing called a job, and they may or may not match on skill level. The messy truth of the workplace, that workers and jobs are deeply interactive: the employee's ability to perform well often depends on his colleagues, how much autonomy his position allows, and the relative rewards for taking risks and playing it safe, is conveniently set aside. It is difficult to explain, let alone fix, macroeconomic factors like weak aggregate demand. Believing that workers don't know how to do jobs right is easy to grasp and, on its surface, easy to remedy: everyone gets more education and training.

The real problem, then, is more appropriately an inflexibility problem. Finding candidates to fit jobs is not like finding pistons to fit engines, where the requirements are precise and can't be varied. Jobs can be organized in many different ways so that candidates who have very different credentials can do them successfully. There are plenty of people out there who could step into jobs with just a bit of training—even recent graduates who don't have much job experience. Despite employers' complaints about the education system, college students are pursuing more vocationally oriented course work than ever before, with degrees in highly specialized fields like pharmaceutical marketing and retail logistics. The real problem, companies don't seem to do on-the-job training anymore. They expect to hire someone and forget about them.

POSITION

It's difficult enough finding a good job to apply to but it's really struggling to find something that fits for you. When you start a new job search, take into consideration the "must have" features of your next position. This can help you narrow down different employment options and allow you to be upfront in interviews about what you are and aren't looking for. Take into consideration your present and future professional plans when launching your search so you're making a choice based on your long-term goals and objectives

When you're graduating and just starting out in the workforce, it may seem that everyone is getting a job faster than you are or no one is moving back home to live with their parents. Well, it's time for a reality check. The truth is that over a million people graduate from college each year, so I promise that whatever your situation, lots and lots of other people are right there with you.

Don't stress about finding the right job right out the door either. Job position changes are common early in a person's working years: Three in four different positions from age 16 to 19, and one to two between 20 and 24.

A positive and upbeat work environment can make all the difference in one's job satisfaction. If you're looking for a certain kind of environment, know the companies you're checking out fit the bill in terms of "feel." Ask to meet with potential colleagues when you interview for a job to get an idea if coworkers share the same attitude and mind-set as you.

But if you are having a difficult time finding that job you want to apply to but you are struggling to find something that fits, try applying to a job that doesn't exist. One of the best ways to create your own position at your company is to assess their needs. Pick a situation that has happened in the recently and show how it could have benefited from your combination of experience and skills.

Write a proposal that outlines the position need you've discovered. Highlight how you will use your skills to resolve the problem and contribute to the immediate objectives of the team or department involved. Then send your proposal to the person who will benefit most from your unique approach.

Without your proactive approach to your career and potential promotion, they may decide to promote one of your peers. By being proactive, you create a win-win situation. You may gain a challenging, enjoyable career opportunity and eliminate the need for a competition. Even if a new career or promotion opportunity does not result from your actions, you have successfully created an opportunity to demonstrate your value to the organization. You have increased the likelihood that they will consider you for the next rewarding career or promotion opportunity.

CAREER GOALS

Many people feel as if they're adrift in the world. They work hard, but they don't seem to get anywhere worthwhile. A key reason that they feel this way is that they haven't spent enough time thinking about what they want from life, and haven't set themselves formal goals. After all, would you set out on a major journey with no real idea of your destination? Probably not!
Goal setting is a powerful process for thinking about your ideal future, and for motivating yourself to turn your vision of this future into reality. The process of setting goals helps you choose where you want to go in life. By knowing precisely what you want to achieve, you know where you have to concentrate your efforts. You'll also quickly spot the distractions that can, so easily, lead you astray.

Career goals are important objectives or milestones people set to evaluate their progress along their career paths. They can be made both by employed people and those searching for jobs, and include things like acquiring training in specialized fields, or determining to reach a certain level of promotion in a set number of years. Though goals can be very useful, they do need to be periodically assessed to ensure that they don't become counterproductive.

People set career goals both before and after they start working. Before a person starts working, he may try to get a certain level of education to become eligible for certain jobs. Someone in a job that he doesn't like may try to get certification in a different area so that he can eventually change jobs. Those in careers that they do like often set time or money-related targets, like working a certain amount of time for a company, or making a specific amount of money. Many people also set goals related to advancement in their company, or for flexibility in their work schedule.

It's usually best to have a mix of ambitions, short-term and long-term as well as specific and general. Long-term goals tend to be more general, since circumstances may change over time, while short-term ones are more specific, since they can be planned for more easily. General career goals are those related to an end, like "become a doctor" or "work from home", while specific ones are related to the steps needed to reach the desired end. If a person wanted to become a doctor, then his first specific goal would be getting good enough grades to get into medical school.

SMART Goals
A useful way of making goals more powerful is to use the SMART mnemonic tool of goal setting. SMART stands for:

S	Specific
M	Measurable
A	Attainable
R	Relevant
T	Trackable

Goal setting is used by top-level athletes, successful business-people and achievers in all fields. Setting goals gives you long-term vision and short-term motivation. It focuses on your acquisition of knowledge, and helps you to organize your time and your resources so that you can make the most of your life. By setting sharp, clearly defined goals, you can measure and take pride in the achievement of those goals, and you'll see forward progress in what might previously have seemed a long pointless grind. You will also raise your self-confidence, as you recognize your own ability and competence in achieving the goals that you've set.

When you've achieved a goal, take the time to enjoy the satisfaction of having done so. Absorb the implications of the goal achievement, and observe the progress that you've made towards other goals. If the goal was a significant one, reward yourself appropriately. All of this helps you build the self-confidence you deserve.

At the start of your career or at any time during your working life, develop your career goals so that you have an idea of where you are going, and have a plan to get there. When you know these two things, you can make the most of your options. Keep in mind that career goals can change as you gain experience, so be prepared to adjust your plan as you go. The following are some tips for setting effective goals.

Express your goals positively
Rather than framing them in terms of what you don't want.

Be precise
Set dates, times, and amount so that you would know when you have achieved your goals.

Set priorities
You need to know which of your goals to focus your attention toward and helps you avoid feeling overwhelmed by having too many goals.

Write your goals down
You need to be visually reminded of them. Write your goals to be precise and clear.

Break down your goals into
You want to be able to get frequent opportunities to accomplish them and feel motivated to take on other goals.

Set realistic goals
You must be able to achieve your goals and know that they are in your own control to do so.

Test your goals
The best way to separate possible goals from impossible ones is to test them, in a modest way, and see what happens.

❦ HEALTHY WORKING ENVIRONMENT ❦

A healthy work environment is critical to the well-being of every workplace. It is essential for the overall satisfaction of employees, for successful recruitment and retention, and for the quality of life. A creating a culture of wellness is paramount, in which all leaders, managers, workers, and ancillary staff have a responsibility as part of a centered team that performs with a sense of professionalism, accountability, transparency, involvement, efficiency, and effectiveness.

But to achieve a healthy work environment, we are often challenged to think differently about our culture, habits and day-to-day practices at work. Change and implementation takes time and effort, and it takes a comprehensive approach that spans physical, cultural, social, and job design conditions.

A good change is offering a flexible workplace. A flexible workplace supports employees to balance work and life commitments. It's an environment in which the workplace culture views this balance as positive and encourages employees to take advantage of options such as:

Flexibility
Flexibility is allowing employees to have the ability to adapt their everyday workday schedule to be able to respond to family issues, such as a child becoming ill, school visits, interviews, or special needs of elders. It typically includes family responsibility leave for employees.

Supportiveness
Having supervisors whose management style values their staff and is characterized by a desire to help employees achieve better work-life balance.

Family Friendly
An overall attitude, belief, and values that support work-family. Creative ideas are options that include maternity, paternity, family and personal leave provisions.

Recognition of Child and Elder Care Needs
Employers providing services that include support for child care, providing access to a service regarding child or elder care, establishing on-site child care or, developing a consortium with other employers in order to provide emergency child care.

Creating a healthy work environment requires the active involvement of employers and employees. Healthy workplace change is a bottom-up and a top-down process. Leadership roles need to be taken by people at all levels of the organization. A healthy organization will create healthy outcomes for its employees through improved health and well-being, and result in reduced costs and improved performance.

Occupational Wellness Assessment

Almost Always = 2 points
Sometimes/Occasionally = 1 point
Very Seldom = 0 points

____ 1. I am happy with my career choice.
____ 2. I look forward to work.
____ 3. My job responsibilities/duties are consistent with my values.
____ 4. The payoffs/advantages in my career field choice are consistent with my values.
____ 5. I am happy with the balance between my work time and leisure time.
____ 6. I am happy with the amount of control I have in my work.
____ 7. My work gives me personal satisfaction and stimulation.
____ 8. I am happy with the professional/personal growth provided by my job.
____ 9. I feel my job allows me to make a difference in the world.
____ 10. My job contributes positively to my overall well-being.

_____ **Total for Occupational Wellness Dimension**

Score: **15 to 20 Points**
Excellent strength in this dimension.

Score: **9 to 14 Points**
There is room for improvement. Look again at the items in which you scored 1 or 0. What changes can you make to improve your score?

Score: **0 to 8 Points**
This dimension needs a lot of work. Look again at this dimension and challenge yourself to begin making small steps toward growth here. Remember: The goal is balanced wellness.

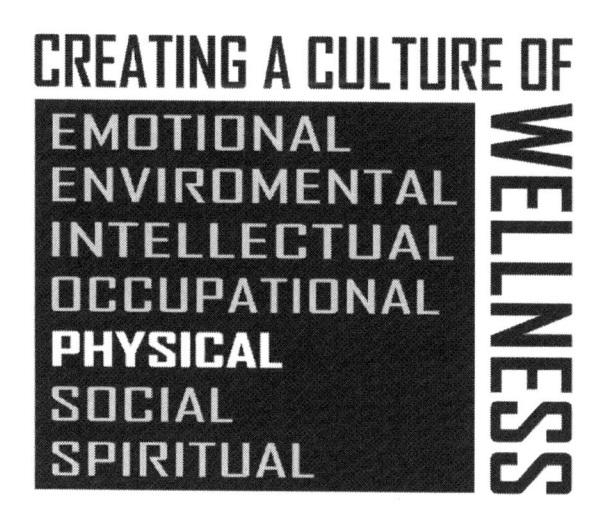

CREATING A CULTURE OF
EMOTIONAL ENVIROMENTAL INTELLECTUAL OCCUPATIONAL **PHYSICAL** SOCIAL SPIRITUAL WELLNESS

Chapter 6

| CHRONIC DISEASE | HEALTH | EXERCISE |
| NUTRITION | WEIGHT MANAGEMENT |

In the busy hustle and bustle of work and family commitments, physical health often gets overlooked, or in some cases even ignored, until there's a problem requiring medical attention. . Health starts in our homes, schools, workplaces, neighborhoods, and communities. We know that taking care of ourselves by eating well and staying active, not smoking, getting the recommended immunizations and screening tests, and seeing a doctor when we are sick all influence our health.

When most people think about health they conjure up images that are related to physical health. Physical health is anything that has to do with our bodies as a physical entity. It has been the basis for active living campaigns and the many eat right fads that have swept our country. A critical part of good physical health is disease prevention. Important first steps to improving physical health. Physical health can be improved in specific ways, even with limited resources. As people take care of their own health needs, they become more able to meet their other physical, educational, emotional, and spiritual needs

Sometimes we expect our bodies to perform these tasks without providing the nourishment and support it needs. But people are living longer than ever before, researchers and policy makers have begun to change the way the they look at health, looking beyond what the causes of death are, but also examine the relationship of health to the quality of life.

You can continue on your current path, the one that lead millions of Americans to health problems, which could have been avoided due to healthier habits or you can invest in your health now. Changing your lifestyle now is the best prevention of chronic diseases, keeping your healthy *and* improve you quality of life.

CHRONIC DISEASE

It has been well documented that as the number of hours worked steadily increases, the level of sedentary nature or low physical activity of the employment role also increases, as does the likelihood of having an inadequate diet. Adults now spend approximately one third of their waking hours at work. Associated with this trend is the alarming growth rate of chronic disease in the community such as obesity, diabetes, heart disease and issues relating to mental health.

There are many contributing factors, however many of the health problems of the workforce are attributable to worsening personal lifestyle choices and the growing levels of workplace stress. Increasing chronic ill health is affecting local and global business performance and national and global economies. Much of this financial burden will be felt by corporations in the form of: absenteeism, presenteeism and lack of productivity both directly and indirectly. Governments, business and individuals all have a role to play in tackling the crisis

More than half of all Americans suffer from one or more chronic diseases. Despite dramatic improvements in therapies and treatment, the rates of disease have risen dramatically. Chronic diseases are ongoing, generally incurable illnesses or conditions, such as heart disease, asthma, cancer, and diabetes. These diseases are often preventable, and frequently manageable through early detection, improved diet, exercise, and treatment therapy.

As a nation, 75% of our health care dollars go to treatment of chronic diseases. These persistent conditions, the nation's leading causes of death and disability, leave in their wake deaths that could have been prevented, lifelong disability, compromised quality of life, and increasing health care costs.

Chronic diseases - such as heart disease, cancer, and diabetes - are the leading causes of death and disability in the United States. And account for over 60% of all deaths in the world. Many chronic diseases could be prevented, delayed, or alleviated, through simple lifestyle changes. The U.S. Centers for Disease Control and Prevention (CDC) estimates that eliminating three risk factors: poor diet, inactivity, and smoking – would prevent:

- ❖ 80% of heart disease and stroke;
- ❖ 80% of type 2 diabetes; and
- ❖ 40% of cancer.

Heart Disease

Heart disease is a broad term used to describe a range of diseases that affect your heart. The various diseases that fall under the umbrella of heart disease include diseases of your blood vessels, such as coronary artery disease; heart rhythm problems heart infections; and heart defects you're born with. The term "heart disease" is often used interchangeably with "cardiovascular disease." Cardiovascular disease generally refers to conditions that involve narrowed or blocked blood vessels that can lead to a heart attack, chest pain (angina) or stroke. Other heart conditions, such as infections and conditions that affect your heart's muscle, valves, or beating rhythm also are considered forms of heart disease. Many forms of heart disease can be prevented or treated with healthy lifestyle choices.

Cancer

Cancer refers to any one of a large number of diseases characterized by the development of abnormal cells that divide uncontrollably and have the ability to infiltrate and destroy normal body tissue. Cancer also has the ability to spread throughout your body. Cancer is the second leading cause of death in the United States. But survival rates are improving for many types of cancer, thanks to improvements in cancer screening and cancer treatment.

<u>Most Common Cancers Found in Men</u>
1) Prostate cancer
2) Lung cancer
3) Colorectal cancer
4) Bladder cancer: White men
Cancer of the mouth & throat: Black men
Stomach cancer: Asian/Pacific Island men

<u>Most Common Cancers Found in Women</u>
1) Breast cancer
2) Lung cancer
3) Colorectal cancer
4) Cancer of the uterus

Diabetes

Diabetes refers to a group of diseases that affect how your body uses blood glucose, commonly called blood sugar. Glucose is vital to your health because it's an important source of energy for the cells that make up your muscles and tissues. It's also your brain's main source of fuel.

Type 1
Various factors may contribute to type 1 diabetes, including genetics and exposure to certain viruses. Although type 1 diabetes typically appears during childhood or adolescence, it also can develop in adults. Despite active research, type 1 diabetes has no cure, although it can be managed. With proper treatment, people who have type 1 diabetes can expect to live longer, healthier lives than they did in the past.

Type 2
With type 2 diabetes, your body either resists the effects of insulin — a hormone that regulates the movement of sugar into your cells — or doesn't produce enough insulin to maintain a normal glucose level. Untreated, type 2 diabetes can be life-threatening. More common in adults, type 2 diabetes increasingly affects children as childhood obesity increases. There's no cure for type 2 diabetes, but you can manage the condition by eating well, exercising and maintaining a healthy weight. If diet and exercise don't control your blood sugar, you may need diabetes medications or insulin therapy.

❦ Health ❦

For a population to be healthy, it must minimize health disparities among segments of the population, including differences that occur by gender, race or ethnicity, education, income, disability, geographic location, or sexual orientation.

Heart disease is the leading cause of death in the United States. Stroke is the third leading cause of death in the United States. Together, heart disease and stroke are among the most widespread and costly health problems facing the Nation today, accounting for more than $500 billion in health care expenditures and related expenses in 2010 alone. Fortunately, they are also among the most preventable.

Controlling risk factors for heart disease and stroke remains a challenge. High blood pressure and cholesterol are still major contributors to the national epidemic of cardiovascular disease. High blood pressure affects approximately 1 in 3 adults in the United States, and more than half of Americans with high blood pressure do not have it under control. The risk of Americans developing and dying from cardiovascular disease would be substantially reduced if major improvements were made across the U.S. population in diet and physical activity, control of high blood pressure and cholesterol, smoking cessation, and appropriate aspirin use.

Diabetes occurs when the body cannot produce or respond appropriately to insulin. Insulin is a hormone that the body needs to absorb and use glucose (sugar) as fuel for the body's cells. Without a properly functioning insulin signaling system, blood glucose levels become elevated and other metabolic abnormalities occur, leading to the development of serious, disabling complications. Diabetes affects an estimated 23.6 million people in the United States and is the 7th leading cause of death. African Americans, Hispanic/Latino Americans, American Indians, and some Asian Americans and Native Hawaiians and other Pacific Islanders are at particularly high risk for the development of type 2 diabetes.

Effective therapy can prevent or delay diabetic complications. However, almost 25 percent of Americans with DM are undiagnosed, and another 57 million Americans have blood glucose levels that greatly increase their risk of developing DM in the next several years. Few people receive effective preventative care, which makes DM an immense and complex public health challenge. Lifestyle change has been proven effective in preventing or delaying the onset of type 2 diabetes in high-risk individuals.

In the past decade, overweight and obesity have emerged as new risk factors for developing certain cancers, including colorectal, breast, uterine corpus (endometrial), and kidney cancers. The impact of the current weight trends on cancer incidence will not be fully known for several decades. Continued focus on preventing weight gain will lead to lower rates of cancer and many chronic diseases. Complex and interrelated factors contribute to the risk of developing cancer. These same factors contribute to the observed disparities in cancer incidence and death among racial, ethnic, and underserved groups. The most obvious factors are associated with a lack of health care coverage and low socioeconomic status.

In the next 15 years, America's senior population will grow by 53 percent. People are living longer lives than ever before. Unfortunately, while we are living longer lives, we are seeing poorer health among people aging into their senior years. Many experience hospitalizations, nursing home admissions, and low-quality care. They also may lose the ability to live independently at home. Chronic health conditions are the leading cause of death among older adults.

Tobacco use is the single most preventable cause of death and disease in the United States. Each year, approximately 443,000 Americans die from tobacco-related illnesses. For every person who dies from tobacco use, 20 more people suffer with at least 1 serious tobacco-related illness. In addition, tobacco use costs the U.S. $193 billion annually in direct medical expenses and lost productivity.

Preventing tobacco use and helping tobacco users quit can improve the health and quality of life for Americans of all ages. People who stop smoking greatly reduce their risk of disease and premature death. Benefits are greater for people who stop at earlier ages, but quitting tobacco use is beneficial at any age.

EXERCISE

Americans are just not as physically active as they were 20 years ago, with the majority of Americans not meeting the daily minimum for physical activity and a very small percentage of those participating in vigorous exercise. As Americans spend more and more time sitting on the job or at home, they spend less time doing physical activity which increases the risk of obesity, diabetes, and other life-threatening cardiovascular diseases.

Physical activity does not have to be formal for it to improve one's health. A physical activity expenditure of 1,000 calories per week has been associated with significant health benefits. This equals to about one hour per day of walking per week. Health benefits also have been recorded for even smaller amounts of exercise for those who are extremely deconditioned or elderly. The American College of Sports Medicine (ACSM) has reported that the incidence of heart attacks is greatest in the habitually inactive individuals. Maintaining physical fitness through regular physical activity has been shown to reduce these risks. There is significant evidence that leading a physically inactive lifestyle may lead to being overweight and even obese. The research shows that even if an overweight or obese adult is unable to achieve the minimum level of physical activity, significant health benefits can be shown by any physical activity and other types of interventions.

Becoming overweight or obese can increase the risk of developing type 2 diabetes. Structured physical activity combined with modest weight loss has been shown to lower the risk of type 2 diabetes by up to 58%. The best results have been attained when combining physical activity with diabetes prevention interventions.

It is also recommended that adults, individuals 18 years and older, engage in moderate-intensity cardiorespiratory exercise for a minimum of 30 minutes at least 5 days a week, for a total of 150 minutes per week. ACSM also recommended that adults should perform strength training 2 to 3 days per week for each of the major muscle groups, which should also include balance, agility, and coordination. The National Strength and Conditioning Association stated that strength training may increase cardiovascular health and reduce health issues associated with cardiovascular disease with a decrease in resting blood pressure, decrease in exercise heart rate, and lowering cholesterol levels, and may assist in the decrease of the risk of type 2 diabetes.

There are barriers associated with participants not living a healthy lifestyle and not obtaining the minimum daily amount of physical activity. These barriers may be one, or a combination of lack of time, lack of energy, fatigue, and health problems. Not only are barriers found internally within the participants but they may also be found within their environment such as presence of hills, lack of street lights, and the lack of sidewalks within a neighborhood or community. Behavior change is a complex process that must begin at an early age. Many can already distinguish healthy from unhealthy wellness behaviors but will not or cannot make the necessary changes to improve their wellness.

🌾 NUTRITION 🌾

Healthy eating is not about strict nutrition philosophies, staying unrealistically thin, or depriving yourself of the foods you love. Rather, it's about feeling great, having more energy, stabilizing your mood, and keeping yourself as healthy as possible—all of which can be achieved by learning some nutrition basics and using them in a way that works for you. You can expand your range of healthy food choices and learn how to plan ahead to create and maintain a tasty, healthy diet

It is easy to grab a hamburger from a fast food restaurant or order a pizza when you are tired and do not feel like cooking. However, eating food high in fat and bad carbohydrates will affect your health in negative ways. Eating a healthy diet may take some getting used to, but it has many benefits for your health.

Most people's lives are so busy these days, they don't think about the health benefits of the foods they put into their mouths. Healthy eating is now something they need to consciously think about because it doesn't come naturally anymore.

Carbohydrates

Carbs are your body's main energy source. And your brain is fueled by carbohydrates. Carbohydrates occur in a variety of forms: simple sugars, more complex starches and fiber. They are found naturally in legumes, grains, vegetables, fruits and milk. They're also added to baked goods and many other foods. Choose healthy carbohydrates and fiber sources, especially whole grains, for long lasting energy. In addition to being delicious and satisfying, whole grains are rich in phytochemicals and antioxidants, which help to protect against coronary heart disease, certain cancers, and diabetes. Studies have shown people who eat more whole grains tend to have a healthier heart. Emphasize natural, nutrient-dense carbohydrates from fruits and vegetables, beans and legumes, and whole grains.

45 to 65% of your total daily calories

Protein

An important nutrient, that is essential for growth and development. Many people eat too much protein. Try to move away from protein being the center of your meal. Focus on equal servings of protein, whole grains, and vegetables. All the cells of your body include protein. Both plant-based and animal-based foods provide protein Emphasize plant sources of protein, such as beans, lentils, soy products and unsalted nuts, they have higher health-enhancing nutrients than are animal sources of protein. Eat seafood twice a week. Meat, poultry and dairy products should be lean or low fat.

10 to 35% of your total daily calories

Fat

Fat is not necessarily bad for you. Dietary fat is a nutrient that helps your body absorb essential vitamins, maintains the structure and function of cell membranes, and helps keep your immune system working. Some types of fat, though, may increase your risk of heart disease and other health problems. Fat also has a lot of calories, increasing the risk of weight gain. Emphasize unsaturated fats from healthier sources, such as lean poultry, fish and healthy oils, such as olive, canola and nut oils.

20 to 35% of your total daily calories

Vitamins & Minerals

Vitamins & Minerals make people's bodies work properly. Although you get vitamins and minerals from the foods you eat every day, some foods have more vitamins and minerals than others. Vitamins fall into two categories: fat soluble and water soluble. The fat-soluble vitamins (A, D, E, and K) dissolve in fat and can be stored in your body. The water-soluble vitamins (C & B-vitamins) need to dissolve in water before your body can absorb them. Minerals are inorganic elements that come from the soil and water and are absorbed by plants or eaten by animals. Your body needs larger amounts of some minerals, such as calcium, to grow and stay healthy. Other minerals like chromium, copper, iodine, iron, selenium, and zinc are called trace minerals because you only need very small amounts of them each day.

The MyPlate illustration shows the five food groups that are the building blocks for a healthy diet using a familiar image, a place setting for a meal. Use this image to think about what goes on your plate or in your cup or bowl for each meal.

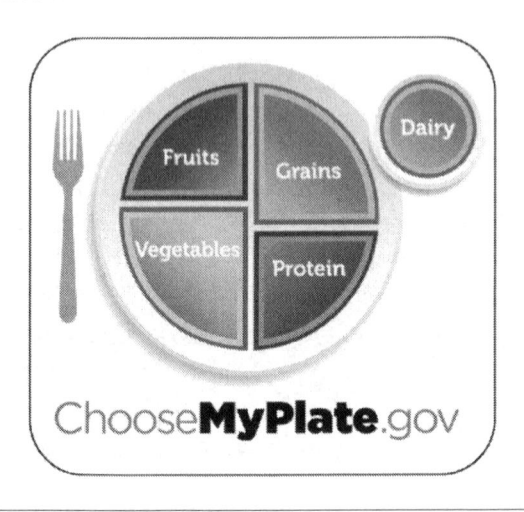

To set yourself up for success, think about planning a healthy diet as a number of small, manageable steps rather than one big drastic change. If you approach the changes gradually and with commitment, you will have a healthy diet sooner than you think.

People often think of healthy eating as an all or nothing proposition, but a key foundation for any healthy diet is moderation. But what is moderation? How much is a moderate amount? That really depends on you and your overall eating habits. The goal of healthy eating is to develop a diet that you can maintain for life, not just a few weeks or months, or until you've hit your ideal weight. So try to think of moderation in terms of balance. Despite what certain fad diets would have you believe, we all need a balance of carbohydrates, protein, fat, fiber, vitamins, and minerals to sustain a healthy body.

For most of us, moderation or balance means eating less than we do now. More specifically, it means eating far less of the unhealthy stuff (refined sugar, saturated fat, for example) and more of the healthy (such as fresh fruit and vegetables). But it doesn't mean eliminating the foods you love. Eating bacon for breakfast once a week, for example, could be considered moderation if you follow it with a healthy lunch and dinner, but not if you follow it with a box of donuts and a sausage pizza. If you eat 100 calories of chocolate one afternoon, balance it out by deducting 100 calories from your evening meal. If you're still hungry, fill up with an extra serving of fresh vegetables.

Healthy eating is about more than the food on your plate, it is also about how you think about food. Healthy eating habits can be learned and it is important to slow down and think about food as nourishment rather than just something to gulp down in between meetings or on the way to pick up the kids.

Make it easy
Instead of being overly concerned with counting calories or measuring portion sizes, think of your diet in terms of color, variety, and freshness. Focus on finding foods you love and easy recipes that incorporate a few fresh ingredients. Gradually, your diet will become healthier and more delicious.

Start slow and create healthy habits
Trying to make your diet healthy overnight isn't realistic or smart. Changing everything at once usually leads to cheating or giving up on your new eating plan. Make small steps, like adding different color vegetables to your diet once a day or switching from butter to olive oil when cooking. As your small changes become habit, you can continue to add more healthy choices to your diet.

<u>Each change in your diet matters</u>
You don't have to be perfect and you don't have to completely eliminate foods you enjoy to have a healthy diet. The long term goal is to feel good, have more energy, and reduce the risk of cancer and disease. Don't let your missteps derail you, every healthy food choice you make counts.

Eating healthy does not mean you have to give help your comfort food. You can enjoy your favorite foods even if they are high in calories, fat or added sugars. The key is eating them less often. Eat smaller portion sizes, or even trying lower-calorie versions. You should also balance them out more physical activity.

Chapter 6 | Physical Wellness

🌾 WEIGHT MANAGEMENT 🌾

Gaining a few pounds during the year may not seem like a big deal, but over the past few years it has become clear that weight is an important health issue. Some people who need to lose weight for their health don't recognize it, while others who don't need to lose weight want to get thinner for cosmetic reasons. Being overweight or obesity may increase the risk of many health problems, including diabetes, heart disease, and certain cancers. If you are pregnant, excess weight may lead to short-term and long-term health problems for you and your child.

Most Americans have tried to eat healthier or be more physically active at some point in their lives. Why, then, do many of us eat high-fat and high-calorie foods and have such a hard time fitting in exercise? You may be wondering: is it even possible to change your habits?

The answer is yes! Change is always possible, and a person is never too out-of-shape, overweight, or old to make healthy changes Old habits die hard. If you want to change your habits, you may find it helpful to make realistic and gradual changes one step at a time and at your own pace. It is important to think about what motivates you, what trips you up, and what you enjoy when it comes to eating and activity habits. There is no such thing as a "one-size-fits-all" approach.

Weight can affect a person's self-esteem. Excess weight is highly visible and evokes some powerful reactions, however unfairly, from other people and the people who carry the excess weight. The amount of weight loss needed to improve your health may be much less than you wish to lose. Your health can be greatly improved by a loss of 5–10% of your weight. That doesn't mean you have to stop there, but it does mean that an initial goal of losing 5–10% of your weight is realistic and valuable.

Talking to your health care provider about your weight is an important first step. Doctors do not always address issues such as healthy eating, physical activity, and weight control during general office visits. It is important for you to bring up these issues to get the help you need. Even if you feel uneasy talking about your weight with your doctor, remember that he or she is there to help you improve your health.

Successful, long-term weight control must focus on your overall health, not just on what you eat. Changing your lifestyle is not easy, but adopting healthy habits may help you manage your weight in the long run. Effective weight-loss programs include ways to keep the weight off for good. These programs promote healthy behaviors that help you lose weight and that you can stick with every day.

Questions to ask your Health Care Provider

- ❖ What is a healthy weight for me?
- ❖ Do I need to lose weight?
- ❖ How much weight should I lose?
- ❖ Could my extra weight be caused by a health problem or by a medicine I am taking?
- ❖ What kind of eating habits may help me control my weight?
- ❖ How much physical activity do I need?
- ❖ How can I exercise safely?
- ❖ Could a weight-loss program help me?

With over 1,000 diet books available on bookstore shelves, popular diets clearly have become increasingly prevalent. At the same time, they have also become increasingly controversial, because some deviate from medical practice or have been criticized by various medical authorities. A comparison of several popular diets showed that at the end of the day, or in this case at the end of the year, sticking with a diet, more than the type of a diet, is the key to losing weight.

Chapter 6 | Physical Wellness

The key, balance your numbers! Observing and recording some aspect of your behavior, such as calorie intake, servings of fruits and vegetables, amount of physical activity, or an outcome of these behaviours, such as weight. Self-monitoring of a behavior usually moves you closer to the desired direction and can produce "real-time" records for review by you and your health care provider. For example, keeping a record of your physical activity can let you and your provider know quickly how you're doing. When the record shows that your activity is increasing, you'll be encouraged to keep it up. Some patients find that specific self-monitoring forms make it easier, while others prefer to use their own recording system.

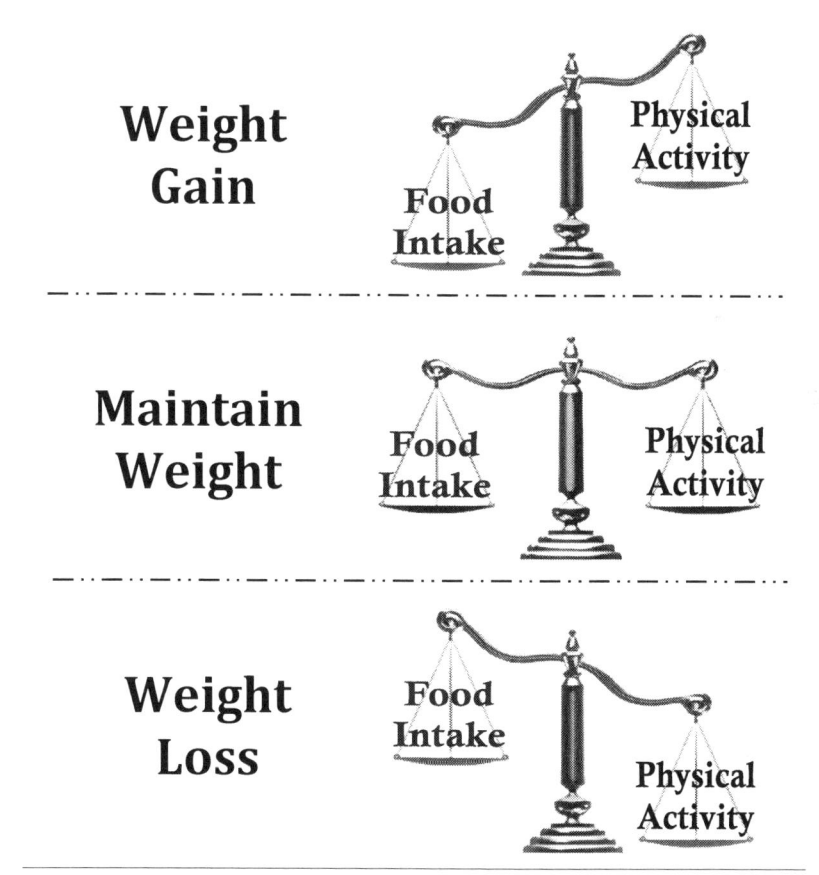

Weight Gain — Food Intake > Physical Activity

Maintain Weight — Food Intake = Physical Activity

Weight Loss — Food Intake < Physical Activity

Physical Wellness Assessment

Almost Always = 2 points
Sometimes/Occasionally = 1 point
Very Seldom = 0 points

____ 1. I exercise aerobically (vigorous, continuous) for 20 to 30 minutes at least three times per week.
____ 2. I eat fruits, vegetables, and whole grains every day.
____ 3. I avoid tobacco products.
____ 4. I wear a seat belt while riding in and driving a car.
____ 5. I deliberately minimize my intake of cholesterol, dietary fats, and oils.
____ 6. I avoid drinking alcoholic beverages or I consume no more than one drink per day.
____ 7. I get an adequate amount of sleep.
____ 8. I have adequate coping mechanisms for dealing with stress.
____ 9. I maintain a regular schedule of immunizations, physicals, dental checkups and self-exams.
____ 10. I maintain a reasonable weight, avoiding extremes of overweight and underweight.

_____ **Total for Physical Wellness Dimension**

Score: **15 to 20 Points**
Excellent strength in this dimension.

Score: **9 to 14 Points**
There is room for improvement. Look again at the items in which you scored 1 or 0. What changes can you make to improve your score?

Score: **0 to 8 Points**
This dimension needs a lot of work. Look again at this dimension and challenge yourself to begin making small steps toward growth here. Remember: The goal is balanced wellness.

CREATING A CULTURE OF

**EMOTIONAL
ENVIROMENTAL
INTELLECTUAL
OCCUPATIONAL
PHYSICAL
SOCIAL
SPIRITUAL**

WELLNESS

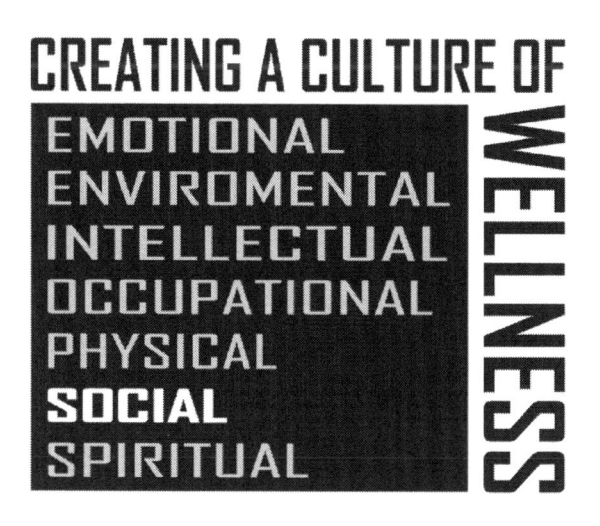

Chapter 7

| FAMILY | FRIENDS | COMMUNITY | CELEBRATION |
| HOSPITALITY | ACCEPTANCE | TOLERANCE |

The social dimension for adults includes being able to create and sustain relationships with, family, friends, peers, and acquaintances over time. Developing appropriate levels of intimacy within those relationships is key for establishing mutual nurturing, feelings of support, camaraderie, and friendship. These are the things that sustain us through life, in good times, and bad. Exhibiting awareness that relationships are dynamic and changing things, that many interests are involved and that successful relationships often call for compromise can help establish trust in a mutual benefit, a ground stone of intimacy. Having the ability to communicate well, address issues that invariably arise within relationships and being able to work through them with friends, family, or significant others represents maturing social behavior. Accepting and giving support, nurturing others as well as letting other people support and care for you also demonstrates social maturity. Also, realizing that there is a legitimate need for fun and leisure time to reconnect with people, recharge the psyche, and invigorate the spirit is very important for our social well-being.

Good social wellness is seen when an individual values the welfare of others and is able to have meaningful and healthy relationships.

🍂 FAMILY 🍂

Family relationships are the foundation of your life. They provide you with some of your greatest growth opportunities as you are challenged to be better parents and spouses. The greatest gifts parents give children is nurturing and caring for them as they grow into adults. In doing so, parents teach children to establish healthy relationships within the family unit and beyond, helping children grow into happy, well-adjusted and successful adults. As life comes full circle, children often have the opportunity to return this gift by caring for their parents as they reach their senior years.

It's no stretch to say that a person has a serious advantage in life if they come from a loving, supportive home. Many people still succeed though they come from less-than-ideal family situations, but having our basic needs met, knowing that our parents love us and learning life lessons at home make all the challenges of day-to-day living that much easier to face. Likely, as an adult you want a happy home for your family.

You want a happy family. But, perhaps, you feel your dreams of family happiness slipping away? You are not alone. It makes you wonder, why is something so universally sought after so hard to achieve? Perhaps we are going about it the wrong way, or perhaps we are working at cross-purposes. You know the old saying, one step forward, take two steps backwards? The reality is that family happiness is not that hard to realize even in today's stressful times. Feeling the security and constancy of love from a spouse, a parent, or a child is a rich blessing. Love is a source of strength and casts out fear. Such love is the desire of every human soul. Here are a few tips on how to manage any future challenges you may face as a family.

Be patient
In love and in parenting, patience is a must. It takes time for people to learn, grow and change. So whether it's you, your spouse or one of your children who is struggling the most, everyone in the family needs to give that person, and the family as a whole, time to grow.

Be creative
You have to be creative when it comes to thinking of new solutions to problems with your spouse or your children. Different things work for different people. So when one strategy doesn't work, try another, until you find the one that works for you.

Be realistic
Marriage and parenthood require a tremendous amount of work. Family life is full of unique challenges, after one developmental stage in the life of a child or a marriage, comes yet another stage. Be realistic about the fact that you are always going to be working on some issue and facing some sort of obstacle.

Maybe you are one of the lucky ones who were raised in a happy and secure family with two loving parents. Maybe you weren't, and growing up was tough without the love and support we longed for. Likely, as an adult you want a happy home for your family. Living peacefully in a family isn't always easy, but marriage and families is the most important social unit. Use these five things to help build a strong and happy family:

Safe Learning Environment
Families are where you learn values, skills, and behavior. Strong families manage and control their learning experiences. They establish a pattern of home life. They select appropriate television programs. They guide their children into the world outside the home. They do not let social forces rule their family life. They involve themselves in neighborhood, school, government, church, and business in ways that support their family values. Strong families teach by example and learn through experience as they explain and execute their values.

Strong Family Bond
Strong families have a sense of loyalty and devotion toward family members. The family sticks together. They stand by each other during times of trouble. They stand up for each other when attacked by someone outside the family. Loyalty builds through sickness and health, want and good fortune, failure and success, and all the things the family faces. The family is a place of shelter for individual family members. In times of personal success or defeat, the family becomes a cheering section or a mourning bench. One also learns a sense of give and take in the family, which helps prepare them for the necessary negotiations in other relationships

Unconditional Love

Love is at the heart of the family. The family is normally the place where love is expressed. It includes privacy, intimacy, sharing, belonging, and caring. The atmosphere of real love is one of honesty, understanding, patience, and forgiveness. Such love does not happen automatically, it requires constant daily effort by each family member. Loving families share activities and express a great deal of gratitude for one another. Love takes time, affection, and a positive attitude.

Humor

It is an escape valve for family tension. Through laughter we learn to see ourselves honestly and objectively. Building a strong family is serious business, but if taken too seriously, family life can become very tense. Laughter balances our efforts and gives us a realistic view of things. To be helpful, family laughter must be positive in nature. Laughing together builds up a family. Laughing at each other divides a family. Families that learn to use laughter in a positive way can release tensions, gain a clearer view, and bond relationships.

Guidance

Family members, usually the adults, must assume responsibility for leading the family. If no one accepts this vital role, the family will weaken. Each family needs its own special set of rules and guidelines. These rules are based on the family members' greatest understanding of one another, not forces. The guidelines pass along from the adults to the children by example, with firmness and fairness. Strong families can work together to establish their way of life, allowing children to have a voice in decision making and enforcing rules.

The best way to begin your discovery of family happiness is to stop looking for it. You already have this pearl in your heart – you just may not realize it. You see, you don't create happiness you discover that it is already yours and then you revel in it. To be a happy family is to share this wisdom and to live in the reveling, together.

🌾 FRIENDS 🌾

Many adults find it hard to develop new friendships or keep up existing friendships. Friendships may take a back seat to other priorities, such as work or caring for children or aging parents. You and your friends may have grown apart due to changes in your lives or interests. Or maybe you've moved to a new community and haven't yet found a way to meet people. Developing and maintaining good friendships takes effort. The enjoyment and comfort friendship can provide, however, makes the investment worthwhile. Understand the importance of friendships in your life and what you can do to develop and nurture friendships. Friends can help you celebrate good times and provide support during bad times. Friends prevent loneliness and give you a chance to offer needed companionship.

Developing and maintaining healthy friendships involves give-and-take. Sometimes you're the one giving support, and other times you're on the receiving end. Letting friends know you care about them and appreciate them can help strengthen your bond. It's as important for you to be a good friend as it is to surround yourself with good friends.

Friends make you feel comfortable with yourself, so you don't need to act like something you're not. Your friends know your shortcomings and love you anyway. You are perhaps the "best version" of yourself when you're with your friends. To that end, a healthy friendship includes plenty of gentle honesty. A friend won't lie to you, but they won't try and hurt your feelings either. As a result, you'll know where you stand with your friend and won't be afraid to share your true opinions.

The false notion that a friend is a friend forever, no matter what, has caused much heartache. All relationships experience ups and downs, and it is important to overlook occasional misunderstandings and differences of opinion. However, if a relationship brings you more pain than pleasure, it is time to reconsider whether or not it is a true friendship and one that should endure. The most important thing to remember is to treat your friends as you would like to be treated. If you do this, your friendships will remain strong and hearty despite issues that may come up.

There's no need to aim for a specific number of friends. Some people benefit from a large and diverse network of friends, while others prefer a smaller circle of friends and acquaintances. There are also different types of friendships. You may have a few close friends you turn to for deeply personal conversations, and more casual friends with whom you see movies, play basketball or share backyard cookouts. Consider what works for you.

Overall, the quality of your relationships is more important than the specific number of friends you have. Above all, stay positive. You may not become friends with everyone you meet, but maintaining a friendly attitude and demeanor can help you improve the relationships in your life and sow the seeds of friendship with new acquaintances.

COMMUNITY

Relationships are the building blocks for all community organizing activities. Whether you want to organize a volleyball game or get rid of more serious issues in your town, you will need lots of good relationships. Why? Because the relationships we have with our coworkers, the communities we serve, and even our adversaries are the means for achieving our goals. People don't work in isolation: we need to be working together! It is our relationships all added together that are the foundation of an organized effort for change. We need lots of people to contribute their ideas, take a stand, and get the work done.

By our very nature, humans are social beings. No one is, as the expression goes, is 'on an island.' We can contribute our positive sense of well-being to our communities of friends, family and colleagues who, through their inspiration and compassion.

Relationships in life are about communities, it's important to engage your personal communities and networks of influence. Your personal community provides you the insights and the support that you need to face the challenges of everyday life and accomplish your goals. Members of your communities will have a shared emotional connection, maybe not with each other but with a common goal or idea. In reality you already have several personal communities.

Cultivating exceptional relationships with others is one of the most courageous, wondrous things you can do. You, paired with another, can be magnificently more than the sum of your parts, especially when the relationship is acknowledged as an extraordinary vehicle for personal growth, profound partnerships and spiritual path.

Community building occurs one-on-one

You need to build relationships with people one-to-one if you want them to become involved in your group or organization. Some people become involved in organizations because they believe in the cause. However, many people become involved in a community group or organization, just because they have a relationship with another person who is already involved.

We need relationships to further our cause
In order to get support from people outside our organizations, we need to build relationships in which people know and trust us.

Relationships give meaning to our lives
We all need a community of people to share the joys and the struggles of organizing and making community change. A little bit of camaraderie goes a long way.

The world has never been more connected, primarily through technology (e.g., Skype, Facebook, Twitter, etc.). The internet and technological advances have transformed the way people communicate and interact with one another. In recent years, new forms of virtual communities that enable people to connect with friends, share interest and activities, build relationships, and collaborate with each other have gained tremendous popularity, and have become the hottest sites on the internet. For many of us, it is now a daily routine to communicate with peers online as it is simpler, and more convenient.

There is always a reason that brings like-minded people together, whatever the means. Recognizing this reason is extremely important, either in knowing how to access it, or perhaps being the catalyst yourself. Life is not about the money or power, but the expression of love to our fellow human, particularly in times of stress. This, after all, is what quality friendships are all about.

🎋 HOSPITALITY 🎋

In today's harried world hospitality is almost a lost art. A beautiful, enriching art that demonstrates that giving is better than receiving. The idea is as old as the creation of mankind. Hospitality is more than a virtuous deed to be checked off a list; it is a mind-set toward life. The word hospitable means receiving guests or strangers warmly and generously; being favorably receptive and open to others. It is letting people into your home and into your life, and its ministry fits our human needs.

Anyone who has experienced this kind of warm reception into a family or a home knows the refreshment it brings the spirit, especially if one is traveling, lonely, or unacquainted in an area.

It seems as though people today do show hospitality towards others, but in a different way than those in previous generations. It may not be custom anymore to provide food, protection, and shelter to a stranger that arrives at someone's door. This could be because there are hotels and restaurants almost anywhere you can go. Hospitality is still shown, however, in modern society.

For example, when someone's car breaks down most people would welcome them into their homes and help them in any way they can without even asking who they are. Also, most people know of someone, be it family or friend, in a different city that would welcome them and provide them with a place to stay and food. Although the hospitality customs of previous generations, there are similarities to them and hospitality is still visible.

Hospitality can be affected by our own selfishness and pride. When we are so wrapped up with our own problems and difficulties, or we wish to jealously preserve what we have and exclude foreigners and strangers from our lives and riches, we are inhospitable. Too much introspection and inwardness will prevent us from truly being present to others. Preoccupation with external appearances, details and activity prevents us from listening and welcoming.

Get in the habit of helping others. While it may not seem necessary, making some time to help other people out regularly will vastly improve your ability to be hospitable. If you are in the habit of rejecting others, you may be inhospitable as a knee-jerk reaction to a situation you are in. A good way to get out of this habit would be to give a dollar to homeless people you see. This may only work for people who live around cities. For anyone else, try to establish at least a weekly routine of doing something like visiting sick people in the hospital. I used to volunteer in a hospital while in high school; believe me, you learn a lot about people who actually do need your help.

ACCEPTANCE

Do you have the heart and a mind that acknowledges, accepts, values, and even celebrates the various ways that people live and interact in the world?

There is a subtle transition that takes place in any culture or society when its constituents go from occasionally living with the less-than-optimal to accepting that this is just the way that things are. And when we begin to regularly accept our failures, we create a culture that anticipates and even rewards or celebrates this failure. People judge other people's color, race, religion, belief, fashion, diet, and just about everything that is different from their own reality. Somehow, this belief of one group, one idea, one faith, or one kind of lifestyle develops a fraternal bond with those whom we see akin to us. However, wars, crimes, and racism emerge from issues of alienation, ostracism, autonomy, and similar forms that manifest desire to be separated, independent, or even simply assertive.

There are very few people in this world who believe that their actions are without reason or justification. Certainly no culture or religion develops a custom just for the hell of it – there's always a purpose. When you come across a cultural or religious difference, your first goal should always be to understand the reasoning behind the purpose to it.

Accepting a cultural or religious difference beyond understands the reasoning at play. Acceptance means that you recognize that this cultural or religious difference is worthwhile and good for the people who practice it.

I'm not suggesting that you accept traditions that are obviously morally wrong to your beliefs, just because another culture says that it's a good thing. Even with more mundane cultural differences though, it's not always a simple jump from understanding the reasoning behind a cultural custom to accepting the cultural custom as a good others. You may think it's just a waste of time. Or that it's a tradition that doesn't solve the problem that is actually at hand, it just distracts from it. We should all strive to understand the cultural differences we come across in our intercultural relationships, even though it may not be possible to accept all cultural differences.

What's important is that the level of acceptance of each other's differences works for your relationship. This means that you're both comfortable with each other's differences, and neither person feels pressured to accept that which that which they find troubling, morally or otherwise.

🌾 TOLERANCE 🌾

Tolerance is respect, acceptance and appreciation of the rich diversity of our world's cultures, our forms of expression and ways of being human. How do democratic, pluralistic societies like the United States, based on religious and cultural tolerance, respond to customs and rituals that may be repellent to the majority? As new groups of immigrants from Asia and Africa are added to the demographic mix in the United States, Canada and Europe, balancing cultural variety with mainstream values is becoming more challenging.

The appreciation of diversity, the ability to live and let others live, the ability to adhere to one's convictions while accepting that others adhere to theirs, the ability to enjoy one's rights and freedoms without infringing on those of others, tolerance has always been considered a moral virtue. Tolerance is also the foundation of democracy and human rights. Intolerance in multi-ethnic, multi-religious or multicultural societies leads to violations of human rights, violence or armed conflict.

Understanding a cultural difference isn't the same as condoning, it is just a way to open up a dialogue with a person from a different background by acknowledging the humanness of their actions and beliefs. If you can't get beyond the "that's nonsense" reaction to a cultural difference, it represents a failure on your part to stretch your mind fully. Of course, that doesn't mean that it's easy to understand the actions and traditions of cultures foreign to us.

Toleration appears to be at risk of being fragmented between various concerns: the demanding claims of identity politics, a concern with the moral and legal limits of toleration, and a new anxiety about sociocultural cohesion or political unity. In the current situation, it seems to be a compromise with few defenders and many detractors.

What we begin to see is a reversal in the opposite direction, towards intolerance. In many countries the contention is now that, in the past, there has been too much leniency, too much accommodation and too little insistence on shared values. Fuelled by anxieties over terrorism, over a lack of 'cohesion' and 'political unity', social disorder and fragmentation along ethnic and religious lines, it is argued that too much tolerance has been afforded to minority groups. That which is tolerated must be consistent with the legitimate rights of others, especially in relation to women and children or freedom of sexual orientation.

Toleration comes to be seen as the cause of pertinent social problems, a sign of weakness or confusion. A new principled intolerance is seen, paradoxically, as necessary to protect the rights of individuals, and the rights, values and the identity of the majority.

Social Wellness Assessment

Almost Always = 2 points
Sometimes/Occasionally = 1 point
Very Seldom = 0 points

____ 1. I contribute time and/or money to social and community projects.
____ 2. I am committed to a lifetime of volunteerism.
____ 3. I exhibit fairness and justice in dealing with people.
____ 4. I have a network of close friends and/or family.
____ 5. I am interested in others, including those from different backgrounds than my own.
____ 6. I am able to balance my own needs with the needs of others.
____ 7. I am able to communicate with and get along with a wide variety of people.
____ 8. I obey the laws and rules of our society.
____ 9. I am a compassionate person and try to help others when I can.
____ 10. I support and help with family, neighborhood, and work social gatherings.

____ **Total for Social Wellness Dimension**

Score: **15 to 20 Points**
Excellent strength in this dimension.

Score: **9 to 14 Points**
There is room for improvement. Look again at the items in which you scored 1 or 0. What changes can you make to improve your score?

Score: **0 to 8 Points**
This dimension needs a lot of work. Look again at this dimension and challenge yourself to begin making small steps toward growth here. Remember: The goal is balanced wellness.

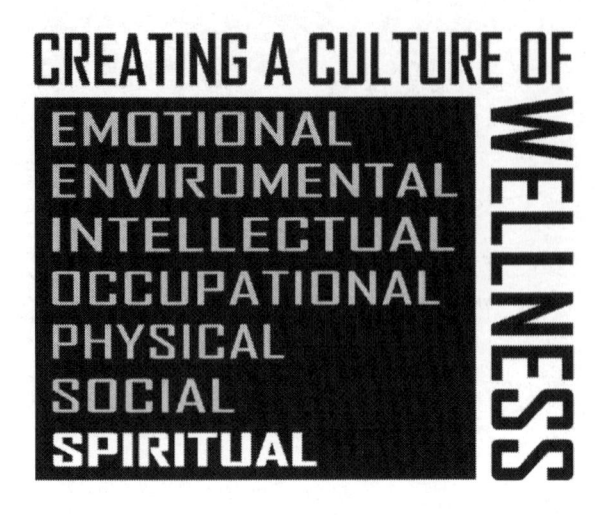

CREATING A CULTURE OF
EMOTIONAL
ENVIROMENTAL
INTELLECTUAL
OCCUPATIONAL
PHYSICAL
SOCIAL
SPIRITUAL
WELLNESS

Chapter 8

| Belief System | Purpose | Core Values |
| Sense of Belonging | Life Satisfaction | Hope |

Many people equate spirituality with a specific religion. Religion and spirituality may exist together, but as Robert Twycross once wrote: "Everyone has a spiritual component, but not everyone is religious." Religion is generally recognized to be the practical expression of spirituality; the organization, rituals and practice of one's beliefs. Religion includes specific beliefs and practices, while spirituality is far broader. Spirituality is thought to include a system of beliefs that encompasses love, compassion and respect for life. Individuals may experience both spirituality and religion very privately within themselves (internally), and/or through social interaction with persons and organizations in an external way.

Spirituality is about our existence, relationships with ourselves, others and the universe. It is something we experience and requires abstract thinking and will. Spiritual development provides us with insight and understanding of ourselves and others. "The spiritual component of a personality is the dimension or function that integrates all other aspects of personhood...and is often seen as a search for meaning in life."

Spiritual wellness for adults involves reflecting upon what inspires and motivates each individual intrinsically. Spiritual wellness encompasses exploring the meanings found in life and uncovering truths, as each person knows them to be. Spirituality is highly individual and can be expressed in many ways. The wellness journey is about discovering how you choose to explore and express your individual self.

Often times this journey involves questioning existence, connecting with people and animals in meaningful ways, developing relationships of faith, sharing one's beliefs, and exchanging energy through thought and deed with other entities within the Universe. Spiritual maturity enables us to find a peaceful co-existence with others who do not share our belief systems. Spiritual commitment encourages us to look for common threads in our beliefs and to celebrate what joins us. Spiritual wellness enables us to come to terms with our existence and order our experiences around our beliefs and goals.

It is a staple of human existence that we feel as though we belong to something or maybe even someone. Given the growing ethnic diversity of the United States, some understanding of the complexities of culture and spirituality is essential for everyone.

❦ BELIEF SYSTEM ❦

The clearer you are about what you value and believe in, the happier and more effective you will be. Beliefs are the assumptions we make about ourselves, about others in the world and about how we expect things to be. Beliefs are about how we think things really are, what we think is really true and what therefore expect as likely consequences that will follow from our behavior.

Your personal belief system is made up of all the previous knowledge, experience and precepts that govern your thoughts, words, behaviour and actions. The current beliefs you possess have developed from an early age, many of which have been acquired through the teachings and learning obtained from parents, teachers, other authority figures and our personal experiences. Having strong beliefs gives us a sense of why we exist and where we are going in life. Our belief system underpins our life purpose and influences our thoughts, values and behaviour

Unlike most belief systems that are less rigid in their external structures, religious beliefs are organized and codified, often based on the teachings and writings of one or more founders of virtually every society that has ever existed. Religious beliefs are of great importance to those who hold them. For thousands of years different religious belief systems have explained how the universe came into existence and appear the way it is, why we are here, how we should live, and what happens when we die.

Religion has provided traditions perpetuated through families and societies are a major factor in developing your belief system. We are often showered with traditions day in and day out when growing up, so they can be extremely easy to adopt, without even questioning. When you believe in a tradition, recognize that they have served some generation well. Yet it does not mean they are based in truth, nor necessarily have continued usefulness for your life.

Organized religion has played the most significant role in the support and propagation of beliefs and faith. This has resulted in an acceptance of beliefs in general. Regardless of how one may reject religion, religious support of supernatural events gives credence to other superstitions in general and the support of faith (belief without evidence), mysticism, and miracles. Most scientists, politicians, philosophers, and even atheists support the notion that some forms of belief provide a valuable means to establish "truth" as long as it contains the backing of data and facts. Belief has long become a socially acceptable form of thinking in science as well as religion. Indeed, once a proposition turns to belief, it automatically undermines opposition to itself.

Your personal belief system can work for you or against you. When it's working against you, your mood is subject to whatever is going on around you. You feel a sense of entitlement. Love is a requirement for your self-esteem. You take things personally or try to control the world around you. You're a perfectionist and nothing is ever good enough. When your personal belief system is working for you, your self-worth is not based on your achievement. You don't seek the approval of others. You're able to find happiness inside yourself. You don't feel entitled to everything. Love is not a requirement for your happiness or self-worth. You don't need other people to agree with you. You let yourself make mistakes and you don't always have to try your best or be the best at everything. You can roll with life's punches and your mind is a fortress that serves and protects you.

> **"Belief creates the actual fact."**
> *- William James -*

Beliefs can also act as barriers towards further understanding. As belief progresses towards faith and dogma, the problems escalate and become more obvious. Religion expresses everything into terms of belief, faith, and absolutes, without need for reason or even understanding. Religion puts reality, morality, love, happiness and desire in a supernatural realm inaccessible to the mind of man.

Parents teach children at a very young age to believe in their personal belief systems. Our parents may not understand the dangers that their beliefs might cause. Our society is preparing future generations to not accept others beliefs, but to honor and fight for their personal ones. This commonly results in conflicts between free expression and censorship. Why not let children develop their own personal belief system beginning at an early age? Letting them identify their own personal sense of purpose.

PURPOSE

Purpose is also called mission, meaning, reason for being, calling, life theme, niche, strategic intent, value added, and business definition. As with vision and values, what labels we use don't matter. As long as we have clear answers to the above questions, we can use whatever terms make sense. We just need to be sure that whatever labels we do use are clear to everybody and used consistently. There's a recurring, consistent pattern in the mission or purpose of most effective leaders, teams, and organizations. That pervasive, underlying theme is, success comes through serving others.

Purpose is your reason, your function and your intention, helping to give you meaning and shape your goals. Purpose is a core principle that both propels you and protects you. It keeps you focused. After all, there are many things you could do, but very few things you SHOULD do.

Like a corporate mission statement, your purpose keeps you on track. Without purpose, people lose their inner spark, their will to live.

List the things that you really enjoy, and why
Add things to the list even if you don't do them now. This list is of your passions, the things that you love to do or do simply for the pleasure they bring you. Being happy in life is you doing the things in life that you were placed here to do.

List the people that you admire, and why
Carefully review the list. Once you review it, look at what you appreciate about others, because that fact is those traits are probably also in you. You are attracted to these qualities and traits because they speak to you. They speak to you because they are a part of your path. Adopt these qualities and traits of others into your daily life. These are your actions.

List things you do without thinking about it
We all have natural talents, most we probably don't even know about. They may be: an eye for detail, a sense of humor, nurturing, focus, or being playful. Consider also, the things you've done that have gotten you into trouble, if you turn them around and look at the positive aspects of it, you'll find a gem of a natural talent that you previously hadn't appreciated. Your natural talents come easily and profoundly, without needing to expend a lot of energy. We all possess unique talents to use in service of our Life Purpose.

Spend time daily on something that you enjoy
By definition, if you're living your life purpose, you will feel exhilarated, excited, happy, and alive. If you're not feeling these things, go back to your lists, and see if there's anything you forgot to write

down, or do the thing that you've been avoiding because you're afraid. You're purpose will guide you through the rough patches.

Finding your purpose is not as hard as most people think. Your purpose is what drives you. It is what makes you passionate. Certainly, you have heard of corporate mission and vision statements. Companies use these statements as directives to help keep business operations on course. It is also a means of succinctly communicating to the world the company's ultimate purpose. This is your opportunity to do the same.

🌾 Core Values 🌾

At the core of spiritual wellness, are values. Values are the standards by which people determine if something is good or bad. Values usually indicate our preferences towards certain things and serve as a guide to what one should do, but not how one should do it. In this area, it is important to know what it is you believe and to be confident in those beliefs.

When you don't know or you haven't clearly defined your personal core values, you end up drifting along in life. You end up trying to fulfill other people's expectations instead of your own. And before you know it, life has passed you by and you haven't even started to live. Instead of basing your decisions on an internal compass, you make choices based on circumstances and social pressures. Trying to be someone else, living without core values is downright exhausting and leaves you feeling empty and shiftless. Living a life in line with your core values brings purpose, direction, happiness, and wholeness.

When you're sure of your core values, decision making becomes much simpler. When faced with a choice, ask yourself: "Does this align with my values?" If it does, you do it. If it doesn't, don't! Instead of freezing up over what's the best thing do to and standing around with you arms up in the air, let your internal compass guide you.

> *"Your beliefs become your thoughts.*
> *Your thoughts become your words.*
> *Your words become your actions.*
> *Your actions become your habits.*
> *Your habits become your values.*
> *Your values become your destiny."*
> *-Mahatma Ghandi -*

Each of us is motivated to move our lives in certain directions. That motivation is determined by the values we subscribe to. Our values are thus the formations and ideations of thought, the distinct formulations of understanding that express what we perceive to be important truths about life. These ideals are then reinforced by our emotions and feelings, which turn those mental perceptions into a vital passion that we hope to realize in our lives. Whether we actually make the effort to implement them is another matter.

Perhaps you have a vague idea about what you value. But if you haven't clearly defined your values, you can end up making choices that conflict with them. And when your actions conflict with your values, the result is unhappiness and frustration. There's something about actually writing down your values that makes you more committed to living them.

In terms of accomplishment, thoughts are mental forms of energy which do not necessarily lead to action. Ideas carry the energy of mental understanding. Opinions carry the force of mental conviction. Attitudes carry the vital force of our emotional endorsement. Values carry the power of psychological commitment and determination. Values issue from a deeper or higher center of motivation in our personalities and therefore carry far greater power than our opinions and attitudes. Personal values are our expressions of emotionalized truths.

SENSE OF BELONGING

In the day of technology it seems all too easy to lose a sense of belonging, to unravel the ties that bind, and to find yourself utterly different and alone. We, as humans, have an instinctive need to belong. The strong sense of belonging stems from the feeling of belonging to a positive social network, family, region, and community. Without these you may become susceptible to loneliness, social anxiety, and depression

All of these factors can influence someone's sense of identity and the extent to which they participate in society. Generally, a strong overall sense of belonging has been show to positively affect self-reported physical and mental health.

Our sense of belonging can emerge from the connections we make with people, places, culture and groups. It can be contextual and we can experience different types of belonging or connection with our family, friends, workplace or community. For a sense of belonging to develop it is necessary that the person experiences a fit or similarity with the people, groups, or places, through mutual or complementary characteristics. Additionally, to build a sense of belonging, people need to have the energy to be involved, the possibility and desire to meaningfully engage, and the potential for shared or complementary values, beliefs or attitudes. To do this, you need to understand:

Quality NOT Quantity
Even if you have hundreds of friends, you will still feel lonely if your relationships with them are not intimate. If you want to get over loneliness then you have to get intimate with some people even if those you choose will be a few in comparison to the number of people you know.

Know Your Needs
Unless you know the type of people you need to form intimate relations with your needs will never be met. You need acceptance from a certain type of people, so acceptance from others that do not fit your personal needs will not help.

Find Your Social Group
The need for belonging can be best fulfilled by having a place in a group setting. Belonging to social groups can give you the same life satisfaction

Religion has traditionally been a powerful force for preserving your sense of community, counteracting the tensions that can easily pull people apart. Most of us have had an experience of a powerful feeling of shared energy and identity among a group of people. Religion offers a sense of knowing one's place with regard to others (one's duties, obligations, and goals) on a broad and sometimes universal scale. For many, religion tells human beings that they are never alone. The structure and communion of religious life provide a consistent sense of belonging.

Of course, some people are going to need closeness, intimacy, attachment, and love with other people more than others. But this much is clear, everyone needs close, caring, intimate relationships marked by emotional depth to live a happy and healthy life. Once you discover that your sense of belonging is the same as everyone else, that you're not lonely and isolated from anyone. You will find the belonging that you need and desire.

🌿 Life Satisfaction 🌿

Satisfaction with one's life is the ultimate goal of us all, yet it seems to remain so elusive. We often hear people talk about "living the dream" and seeking more "life satisfaction and happiness". People have, and continue to search for, satisfaction with their lives. But happiness and life satisfaction are quite separate things. Happiness is a positive emotional state which can occur at any given point in time.

Life satisfaction, on the other hand, is more representative of how someone feels about their whole life, as well as where life is heading in the future. For many people this is a difficult question to answer fully. Knowing what we truly want in life and what would truly make us feel happy and satisfied is not something we ask ourselves enough. Spending time to reflect on our lives, including past, present and future can be a really useful tool in working towards life satisfaction which, in turn, brings with it more happiness.

It is found that religious people tend to be more satisfied with their lives than nonbelievers with the establishment of closer ties to their neighbors and building social networks within their congregation. Church friendships seem to involve something that lifts life satisfaction even more. Religion offers people to spend doing things they find most meaningful, are most competent at, and are able to take the most pleasure in it.

Life satisfaction gets better when we get older. Why? It may be because as we age we come to realize that most of the important things in life are not for sale. Among these are our time, work satisfaction, friendship, and pleasures of solitary thought, reading, and other forms of non-commercial leisure. Life satisfaction is the ultimate goal that we as human beings are striving to achieve our entire lives. Why should it take so long to realize that the best things in life are not sold?

🌿 Hope 🌿

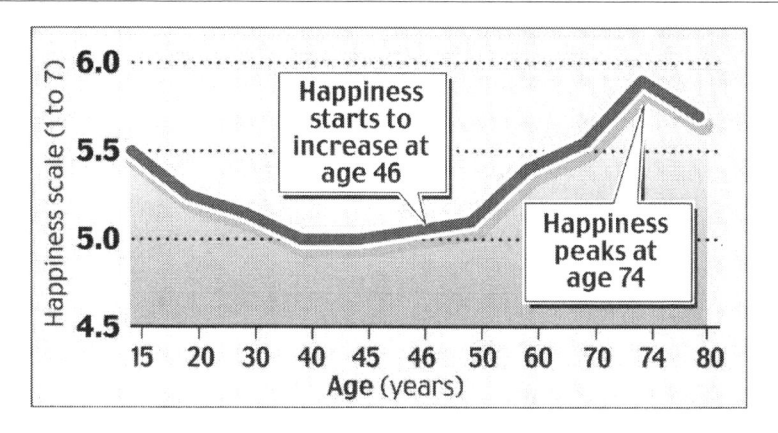

Listen to any religious speaker and you are sure to hear the words hope and faith. Even within self-help circles these words and thrown around and used on a regular basis. Most people will use hope and faith interchangeably, but the two words are different and we all should have them within our vocabulary. More importantly, we should know what these words mean and how they affect us and our ability to create and live the life of our dreams. Few people ever take the time to understand the power of the words they use, and how those words relate to them.

Hope is a portion or part of faith. Faith and hope, in my mind, are overlapping realities: hope is faith in the future tense. So... most of faith is hope.

Hope is powerful word that we must all learn to use. In order to have faith and start looking for a path to follow we must first have hope. Hope is a driving force that things will be better, that things can be better. Hope gives us purpose. To hope is to believe, trust, or maybe desire a certain outcome. People are passionately hopeful regarding different subjects. Every living, breathing, functioning being carries a certain degree of hope. But it is this hope in itself that keeps our hearts pumping, our spirits lifted, and our heads held high. And yes, lost hope can cause more pain and suffering than we often give credit for.

Many of us have a tendency to focus on the negative side of our circumstances. But we can change that attitude, nothing is ever hopeless. Hope is about joyfully looking forward to change for the better, refusing to give up.

Without hope, every day becomes a challenge. The cup is no longer half full-it's half empty. It is at this point that attitude and perspective will either make or break a person. Life is difficult. There are many obstacles. Having goals is not enough. One has to keep getting closer to those goals, amidst all the inevitable twists and turns of life. Hope allows people to approach problems with a mindset and strategy-set suitable to success, thereby increasing the chances they will actually accomplish their goals.

As we lose hope, we tend to lose focus. Our needs and wants are not being met. You must recognize all you have to be thankful for, all your worries will begin to seem less like problems and more like opportunities. Take these opportunities to grow, to change, and to make change. By no means am I saying you will live a life free from any imperfection.

Learn to love imperfections, whatever they may be. Love the people who push your buttons. Maybe you crossed paths with these people so that they may learn a lesson or two from you. Where ever you go, go with unyielding faith. Hope that the choices you are making are, in fact, the right ones. If you strive for what is right, there is no time for shame, regret, or guilt. Only make time for growth. Love unconditionally and above all, remain hopeful.

If you don't believe in what you're doing, nothing that great will happen. By contrast, when you have a bit of hope, and when you can get yourself to act on it, to put yourself out there in a way that you might not normally do, a lot of good things are likely to happen. If you come through and succeed, you start to believe more in what you're doing, which in turn grows the odds of you being successful and ultimately increases your hope. Put simply, hope involves the will to get you there, and the different ways to get you there.

Spiritual Wellness Assessment

Almost Always = 2 points
Sometimes/Occasionally = 1 point
Very Seldom = 0 points

____ 1. I feel comfortable and at ease with my spiritual life.
____ 2. There is a direct relationship between my personal values and daily actions.
____ 3. When I get depressed or frustrated, my spiritual beliefs and values give me direction.
____ 4. Prayer, meditation, and/or quiet personal reflection is/are important in my life.
____ 5. Life is meaningful for me, and I feel a purpose in life.
____ 6. I am able to speak comfortably about my personal values and beliefs.
____ 7. I am consistently striving to grow spiritually and I see it as a lifelong process.
____ 8. I am tolerant of and try to learn about others' beliefs and values.
____ 9. I have a strong sense of life optimism and use my thoughts and attitudes in life-affirming ways.
____ 10. I appreciate the natural forces that exist in the universe.

____ **Total for Spiritual Wellness Dimension**

<u>Score: **15 to 20 Points**</u>
Excellent strength in this dimension.

<u>Score: **9 to 14 Points**</u>
There is room for improvement. Look again at the items in which you scored 1 or 0. What changes can you make to improve your score?

<u>Score: **0 to 8 Points**</u>
This dimension needs a lot of work. Look again at this dimension and challenge yourself to begin making small steps toward growth here. Remember: The goal is balanced wellness.

HELPFUL INFORMATION

PERSONAL VALUES CHECKLIST

Physical Values	Interpersonal Values	Psychological Values
Accuracy	All for One & One for All	Adventurousness
Beauty	Concern for Others	Commitment
Cleanliness	Equality	Creativity
Content over Form	Collaboration	Decisiveness
Continuous Improvement	Cooperation	Determination
Discipline	Coordination	Equanimity
Efficiency	Community	Faith
Endurance	Fairness	Goodwill
Excellence	Freedom	Goodness
Hard Work	Harmony	Gratitude
Maximum Utilization of Resources	Honesty	Integrity
Orderliness	Loyalty	Knowledge
Perfection in Details	Pleasing Others	Love
Punctuality	Respect for Others	Openness
Quality of Work	Self-Giving	Perseverance
Regularity	Service to Others	Personal Growth
Safety	Teamwork	Resourcefulness
Speed	Tolerance	Self-Reliance
Systemization	Trust	Self-Respect
		Truth

SETTING S.M.A.R.T. GOALS

Specific
State exactly what you want to accomplish.

_____

_____

_____

Measurable
How will you determine if you completed your goal(s)?

_____

_____

_____

Attainable
Can you actually do something to make it happen? If so, how?

_____

_____

_____

Relevant
Is your goal relevant to you living a happier & healthier lifestyle?

_____

_____

_____

Timetable
Set target completion dates for each task(s) that will get you towards you goal(s)

_____

_____

_____

YOUR WELLNESS PROFILE

Fill in your strengths for each dimension. Once you've completed your lists, choose your five most important strengths, and circle them. Use your strengths to build on your weaknesses.

Emotional	Physical

Environmental	Social

Intellectual	Spiritual

Occupational

ESTIMATED NUMBER OF STEPS TO WALK A MILE BASED ON GENDER, HEIGHT, & PACE

		MEN				WOMEN		
HEIGHT	20 Minute Mile	18 Minute Mile	16 Minute Mile	14 Minute Mile	20 Minute Mile	18 Minute Mile	16 Minute Mile	14 Minute Mile
5'0	2340	2213	2149	2086	2371	2244	2117	1991
5'1	2326	2199	2135	2072	2357	2230	2103	1977
5'2	2311	2184	2120	2057	2343	2216	2089	1962
5'3	2297	2170	2106	2043	2329	2216	2075	1948
5'4	2282	2155	2091	2028	2315	2216	2061	1933
5'5	2268	2141	2077	2014	2301	2216	2047	1919
5'6	2253	2127	2063	1999	2287	2216	2033	1904
5'7	2253	2127	2063	1985	2273	2216	2019	1890
5'8	2253	2127	2063	1970	2259	2216	2005	1875
5'9	2253	2127	2063	1956	2245	2216	1991	1861
5'10	2253	2127	2063	1941	2231	2216	1977	1846
5'11	2253	2127	2063	1927	2217	2216	1963	1832
6'0	2253	2127	2063	1912	2203	2216	1949	1817
6'1	2253	2127	2063	1898	2189	2216	1935	1803
6'2	2253	2127	2063	1883	2175	2216	1921	1788
6'3	2253	2127	2063	1869	2161	2216	1907	1774
6'4	2253	2127	2063	1854	2147	2216	1893	1759
6'5	2253	2127	2063	1840	2133	2216	1879	1745
6'6	2253	2127	2063	1825	2119	2216	1865	1730
6'7	2253	2127	2063	1811	2105	2216	1851	1716

POSSIBLE HEALTH RISK BASED OFF OF YOUR BODY FAT PERCENTAGE BASED OFF AGE

BODY FAT %	MEN ≤19	MEN 20-29	MEN 30-39	MEN 40-59	MEN ≥50	WOMEN ≤19	WOMEN 20-29	WOMEN 30-39	WOMEN 40-59	WOMEN ≥50	
≤3 – 12											ELEVATED RISK
13 – 19											HEALTHY
20 – 26											LOW RISK
27 – 31											ELEVATED
32 – 39											HIGH RISK
≥40											SEVERELY HIGH RISK

Chapter 9 | Helpful Information

THE RECOMMENED DIET AS A PERCENTAGE OF YOUR DAILY CALORIE INTAKE

CARBOHYDRATES   **45-65%**
  SIMPLE   LESS THAN 25%
  COMPLEX   20%-40%

PROTEIN   **10-35%**

FAT   **20-35%**
  MONSATURATED   UP TP 20%
  POLYSATURATED   UP TO 10%
  SATURATED   LESS THAN 7%

CHOLESTEROL GUIDELINES

TOTAL CHOLESTEROL
  DESIRABLE   LESS THAN 200 mg/dL
  ELEVATED HEALTH RISK   200 - 239 mg/dL
  HIGH HEALTH RISK   OVER 240 mg/dL

LDL CHOLESTEROL
  DESIRABLE   LESS THAN 100 mg/dL
  SLIGHT HEALTH RISK   100 - 129 mg/dL
  ELEVATED HEALTH RISK   130 - 159 mg/dL
  HIGH HEALTH RISK   160 - 189 mg/dL
  VERY HIGH HEALTH RISK   OVER 290 mg/dL

HDL CHOLESTEROL
  HIGH HEALTH RISK   LESS THAN 40 mg/dL
  ELEVATED HEALTH RISK   40 - 59 mg/dL
  DESIRABLE   OVER 60 mg/dL

GLUCOSE GUIDELINES

NORMAL   LESS THAN 100 mg/dL
PRE-DIABETES   101-125 mg/dL
DIABETES   OVER 126 mg/dL

BLOOD PRESSURE GUIDELINES

	SYSTOLIC	*DIASTOLIC*
NORMAL	LESS THAN 120	LESS THAN 80
PRE-HYPERTENSION	121-139	81-89
HIGH BLOOD PRESSURE	140-159	90-99
SEVERELY HIGH BLOOD PRESSURE	160+	100+

BLOOD PRESSURE LOG

DAY / TIME	*BLOOD PRESSURE*	*HEART RATE*

Chapter 9 | Helpful Information

DAILY FOOD JOURNAL	
DAY:	**DATE:**
BREAKFAST	
LUNCH	
DINNER	
SNACKS	
DRINKS *(water, coffee, soda, alcohol)*	
NOTES:	

DAILY FOOD JOURNAL	
DAY:	**DATE:**
BREAKFAST	
LUNCH	
DINNER	
SNACKS	
DRINKS *(water, coffee, soda, alcohol)*	
NOTES:	

Chapter 9 | Helpful Information

WEEKLY MEAL PLAN

Monday

Tuesday

Wednesday

Thursday

Friday

Saturday

Sunday

GROCERY LIST

☐	☐	☐
☐	☐	☐
☐	☐	☐
☐	☐	☐
☐	☐	☐
☐	☐	☐
☐	☐	☐
☐	☐	☐
☐	☐	☐
☐	☐	☐
☐	☐	☐
☐	☐	☐

Chapter 9 | Helpful Information

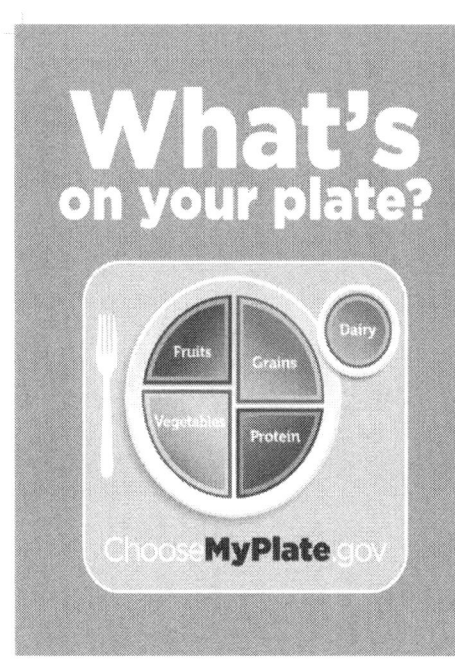

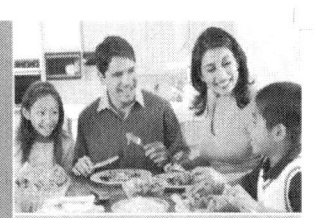

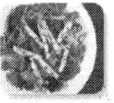

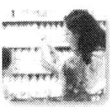

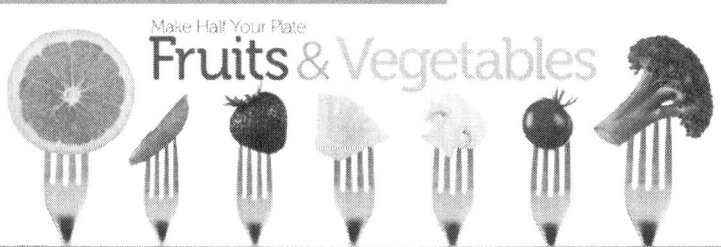

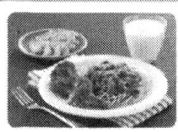

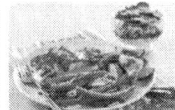

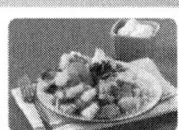

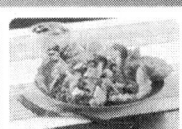

DAY 1

BREAKFAST
Creamy Oatmeal (Cooked in Milk)
½ cup uncooked oatmeal
1 cup fat-free milk
2 tbsp raisins
2 tsp brown sugar
Beverage: 1 cup orange juice

LUNCH
Taco Salad
    2 oz tortilla chips
    2 oz cooked ground turkey
    ¼ cup kidney beans
    ½ oz low-fat Mexican blend cheese
    ½ cup chopped lettuce
    ¼ cup avocado
    1 tsp lime juice
    2 tbsp salsa
Beverage: 1 water or unsweetened tea

DINNER
Personal Spinach Lasagna
    1 cup cooked lasagna noodles
    ½ cup spinach
    ½ low-fat ricotta cheese
    1 oz skim mozzarella cheese
    ½ cup tomato sauce
1 whole wheat roll
Beverage: 1 cup orange juice

SNACKS
2 tbsp raisins
1 oz unsalted almonds

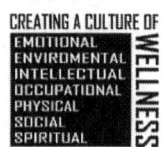

Sample Daily 2,000 Calorie Menu

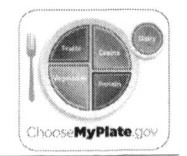

CREATING A CULTURE OF
EMOTIONAL
ENVIRONMENTAL
INTELLECTUAL
OCCUPATIONAL
PHYSICAL
SOCIAL
SPIRITUAL
WELLNESS

ChooseMyPlate.gov

DAY 2

BREAKFAST
Breakfast Burrito
 1 8" flour tortilla
 1 scrambled egg
 ¼ cup black beans
 2 tbsp salsa
1 large grapefruit
Beverage: 1 cup fat free chocolate milk

LUNCH
Tuna Salad Sandwich
 2 slices rye bread
 2 oz tuna
 1 tbsp mayonnaise
 1 tbsp chopped celery
Beverage: 1 cup water or unsweetened tea

DINNER
Baked Salmon on Beet Greens
 4 oz salmon
 1 tsp olive oil
 2 tsp lemon juice
 ½ cup cooked beet greens
Quinoa with Almonds
 ½ cup quinoa
 ½ oz slivered almonds
Beverage: 1 cup water or unsweetened tea

SNACKS
1 cup frozen yogurt

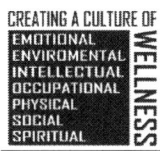

Sample Daily 2,000 Calorie Menu

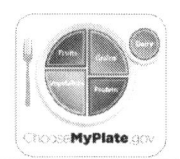

Chapter 9 | Helpful Information

DAY 3

BREAKFAST
French Toast
  2 slices whole wheat bread
  3 tbsp fat-free milk
  1 egg
  2 tsp margarine
  1 tbsp real maple syrup
½ grapefruit
Beverage: 1 cup fat-free milk

LUNCH
Turkey Sandwich
  1 whole wheat pita bread
  3 oz sliced turkey
  2 sliced tomatoes
  ¼ cup chopped lettuce
  1 tsp mustard
  1 tbsp mayonnaise
  ½ cup grapes
Beverage: 1 cup tomato juice

DINNER
Steak and Potatoes
  4 oz broiled beef steak
  ¾ cup mashed potatoes
  ½ cup cooked green beans
  1 tsp margarine
  1 tsp honey
1 whole wheat roll
Beverage: 1 cup water or unsweetened tea

SNACKS
1 cup non-fat fruit yogurt

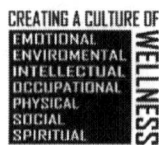

Sample Daily 2,000 Calorie Menu

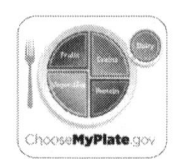

CREATING A CULTURE OF
EMOTIONAL
ENVIRONMENTAL
INTELLECTUAL
OCCUPATIONAL
PHYSICAL
SOCIAL
SPIRITUAL
WELLNESS

ChooseMyPlate.gov

Healthy Recipe Substitutions

1lb Ground Beef	1lb Ground Turkey
1oz Cheddar, Swiss, or American Cheese	1oz skim Mozzarella, or any low- fat cheese
1 Egg	2 Egg Whites
1 cup Whole Milk	1 cup Skim Milk
1 cup Cream	1 cup Evaporated Skim Milk
1 cup Sour Cream	1 cup Greek Yogurt
1oz Chocolate	3tbsp Cocoa Powder in 1tbsp Peanut Oil
1 cup Sugar	1 cup Apple Sauce
1 cup Oil or Butter	1 cup Apple Sauce
1 cup Sugar	2tbsp Stevia
½ cup Ice Cream	½ cup Frozen Yogurt
2tbsp Syrup	2tbsp Pureed Fruit
Seasoned Salt	Fresh Herbs

PERSONAL EXERCISE LOG

1) WARM UP   (5x -7x PER WEEK)

EXERCISE	TIME	INTENSITY

2) CARDIO WORKOUT   (5x -7x PER WEEK)

EXERCISE	TIME	INTENSITY

3) COOL DOWN   (5x -7x PER WEEK)

EXERCISE	TIME	INTENSITY

4) STRENGTH TRAINING   (2x-3x PER WEEK)

EXERCISE	SETS	REPS	WEIGHT	REST

5) STRETCHING   (5x -7x PER WEEK)

EXERCISE	SETS	TIME TO HOLD STRETCH

SAMPLE WORKOUT FOR A HEALTHY INDIVIDUAL TO DO AT HOME

1) WARM UP (5x -7x PER WEEK)

EXERCISE	TIME	INTENSITY
LIGHT WALKING	3-5 MINUTES	LOW

2) CARDIO WORKOUT (5x PER WEEK)

EXERCISE	TIME	INTENSITY
WALKING	25-35 MINUTES	MEDIUM / HIGH

3) COOL DOWN (5x PER WEEK)

EXERCISE	TIME	INTENSITY
LIGHT WALKING	3-5 MINUTES	LOW

4) STRENGTH TRAINING (3x PER WEEK)

EXERCISE	SETS	REPS	WEIGHT	REST
SQUAT WITH ALTERNATING LEG KICK	2	20	BODY WEIGHT	30 SECONDS
STANDING CALF RAISE	2	20	BODY WEIGHT	30 SECONDS
WALL PUSH-UP	2	12	BODY WEIGHT	30 SECONDS
SEATED BACK EXTENSIONS	2	12	BODY WEIGHT	30 SECONDS
BICEPS CURL-TO-SHOULDER PRESS	2	20	BODY WEIGHT	30 SECONDS
STANDING LATERAL LEG LIFT	2	15	BODY WEIGHT	30 SECONDS
SEATED LATERAL ARM RAISE	2	25	BODY WEIGHT	30 SECONDS

5) STRETCHING (3-5x PER WEEK)

EXERCISE	SETS	TIME TO HOLD STRETCH
REAR SHOULDER STRETCH	1	30 SECONDS
TRICEPS STRETCH	1	30 SECONDS
SEATED HAMSTRING STRETCH	1	30 SECONDS
STANDING CALF STRETCH	1	30 SECONDS

Chapter 9 | Helpful Information

DETERMINING YOUR TARGET EXERCISE HEART RATE ZONES

220 − Your Age = _____
Max Heart Rate (MHR)

Low Intensity	Medium Intensity	High Intensity
____ x .60 = MHR ____ +/- 5 Exercise Heart Rate Exercise Heart Rate Zone ____ - ____	____ x .70 = MHR ____ +/- 5 Exercise Heart Rate Exercise Heart Rate Zone ____ - ____	____ x .85 = MHR ____ +/- 5 Exercise Heart Rate Exercise Heart Rate Zone ____ - ____

------------- **EXAMPLE** -------------

** 57 YEARS OLD **

220 − **57** = **163**
Max Heart Rate (MHR)

Low Intensity	Medium Intensity	High Intensity
163 x .60 = MHR **98** +/- 5 Exercise Heart Rate **Low Intensity** Exercise Heart Rate Zone **93** - **103**	**163** x .70 = MHR **114** +/- 5 Exercise Heart Rate **Medium Intensity** Exercise Heart Rate Zone **109** - **119**	**163** x .85 = MHR **138** +/- 5 Exercise Heart Rate **High Intensity** Exercise Heart Rate Zone **133** - **143**

Made in the USA
San Bernardino, CA
12 January 2016